MENSA®
BRAIN
BENDERS

FOR SENIORS

100

LARGE PRINT PUZZLES AND ACTIVITIES TO KEEP YOUR MIND SHARP

DAVID MILLAR
WITH AMERICAN MENSA

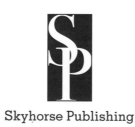

Skyhorse Publishing

Skyhorse Publishing books may be purchased in bulk at special discounts for sales promotion, corporate gifts, fund-raising, or educational purposes. Special editions can also be created to specifications. For details, contact the Special Sales Department, Skyhorse Publishing, 307 West 36th Street, 11th Floor, New York, NY 10018 or info@skyhorsepublishing.com.

Skyhorse® and Skyhorse Publishing® are registered trademarks of Skyhorse Publishing, Inc.®, a Delaware corporation.

Visit our website at www.skyhorsepublishing.com.

10 9 8 7 6 5 4 3 2 1

Library of Congress Cataloging-in-Publication Data is available on file.

Interior design and layout by Chris Schultz
Cover design by Kai Texel
Cover image by Getty Images

ISBN: 978-1-5107-7886-3

Printed in China

Contents

Acknowledgments

This book is dedicated to Jennifer Loyd, who helps me care for my brain when I'm not busy using it to write puzzles.

Thanks to my test-solvers:

- Aurath
- Zach Barnett
- Colleen Coughlin
- Nancy Coughlin
- Kal-el Dwight
- Jack Martin
- Margot Schuh
- Shawn VanNortrick
- wen
- William Zambole

. . . and thank you for solving!

Dave Millar

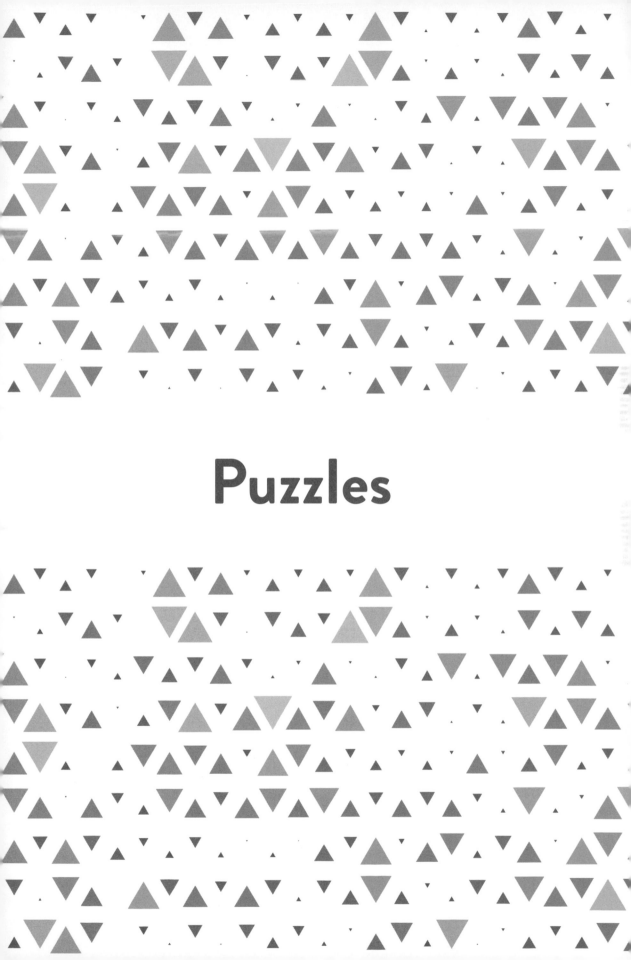

Puzzles

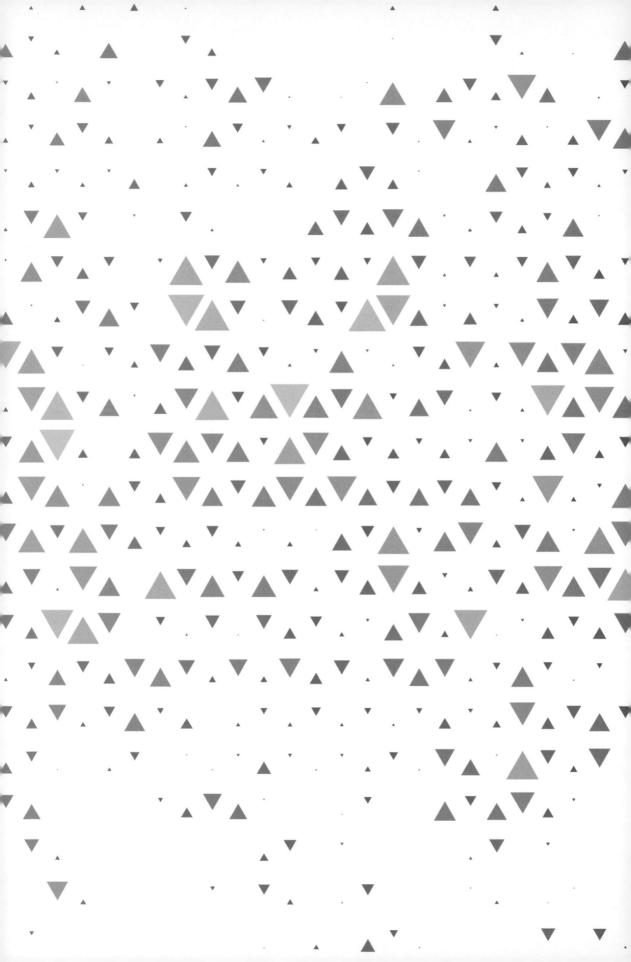

Rows Garden 1

Using the clues provided, enter a letter into each triangle to fill the garden. Each row contains one or two entries, and each hexagonal flower contains a six-letter word wrapped around the center. It's up to you to determine where to place the starting letter and the direction of the word.

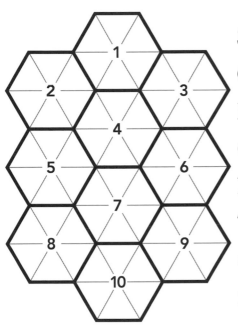

Something on VHS?

Cartoon bear / When pigs fly

Faithful / Traditional pizzelle flavor

Orb / Eye part

Number of "wonders" / Affirmations

Take out / Run with purpose

Color slightly / Maslow's interests

Sick

Flowers

1. Heavenly
2. Dairy product
3. Improve
4. Some stuffed "babies"
5. Cold weather gear
6. "Affirmative"
7. A house of Congress
8. Eye part
9. Kept
10. Legume

Cube Logic 1

Which of the two templates can be folded to produce the exact same block?

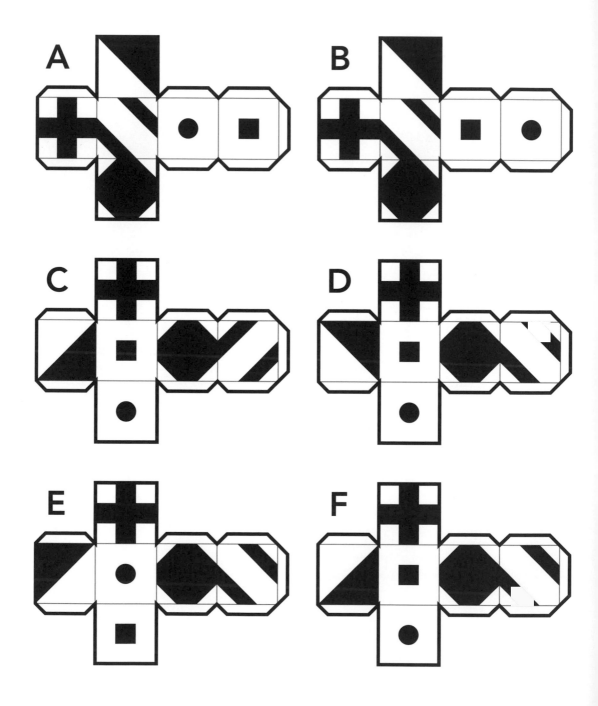

Sudoku TV 1

Place one of each unique letter from HAPPY DAYS into each row, column, and 2 × 3 block.

H					S
	A	P			
			P	Y	
					D
	D	A	Y	S	
		S			

Woven Words 1

Use the clues to weave six words together in the grid below; three going across and three going down. The unwoven letters have been placed to get you started.

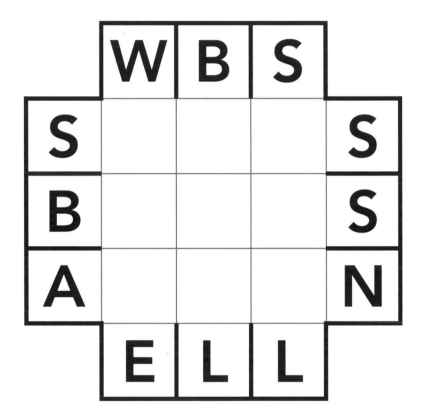

Flight-related

Items on a field

An herb

Stadium contents

Take

Apropos hair piece

Rearrangement 1 & 2

Rearrange the letters in CHILDREN DO SOLO to spell a place with fifties vibes where the kids might get their own menu.

Rearrange the letters in HAIRPIN GIFTS to spell an activity where you might make do with a hairpin if you forgot a hook.

Penny Candy 1

Penny candy has gone up in price a fair bit. Use the total prices of the sets of four candies to figure out how much each piece of candy costs.

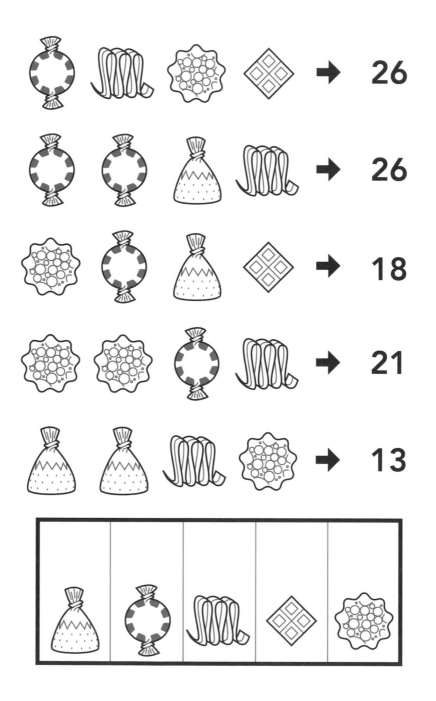

Word Funnel 1

Fill each section of the funnel with a six-letter word made up of the six letters above it. Clues have been provided in no particular order.

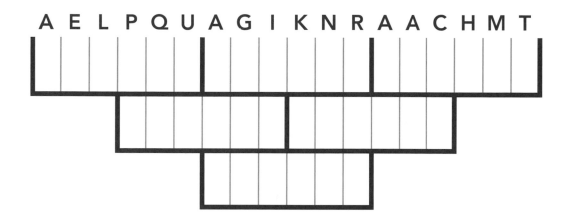

A E L P Q U A G I K N R A A C H M T

Member of a particular religious sect

Place of business

Making animals more friendly

Green tea powder

Proud display

Cleaning up during fall

Chess Sum Sudoku 1

Place a digit from 1 to 5 into each empty cell so that each row, column, and 2 × 3 block contains each digit once, without repetition. The chess knights in the grid display the sum of the digits in the cells which they can attack.

Throwing Shade 1

Shade some cells so the remaining letters in each row and column spell answers to the provided clues. Clues are sorted alphabetically by answer.

P	S	O	H	L	A	R	P	A
A	G	R	L	E	N	R	A	E
U	D	U	D	P	U	A	R	L
S	T	T	U	M	M	P	S	S
H	A	A	I	A	R	E	P	A
R	U	H	N	I	E	T	T	O
P	R	N	M	O	D	O	H	N
L	A	G	E	N	O	O	N	E
E	D	E	U	K	A	R	P	L

Rows

- Location
- Beloved
- Paired
- Actor Wilder
- Angelic instrument
- Midday
- Energy type
- Tree remnants
- Golden Rule word

Columns

- A tree
- A snake type
- Glow
- Sand mass
- Citrus fruit
- Solo
- A color
- Type of dinosaur
- Handsome fella

Cube Logic 2

Which of the two templates can be folded to produce the exact same block?

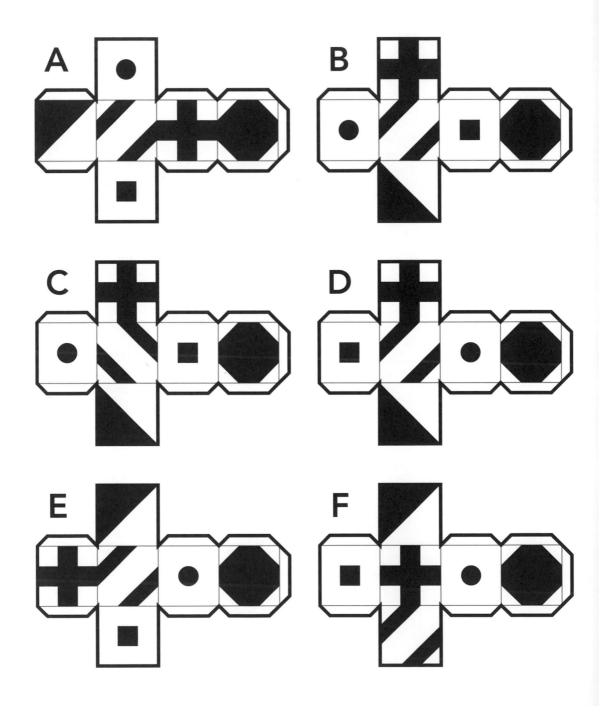

NO Uncertain Terms 1

These uncertain terms have had all their letters removed except for NO. Ascertain the pairings of blanks and clues, and fill the blanks to form the answers.

_ _ _ N O _

_ _ N O _

_ N O _ _ _

_ _ N O

N O _ _ _ _

A type of rowboat

An adequate amount

A posted warning

A small fish

A popular city in Nevada

Woven Words 2

Use the clues to weave six words together in the grid below; three going across and three going down. The unwoven letters have been placed to get you started.

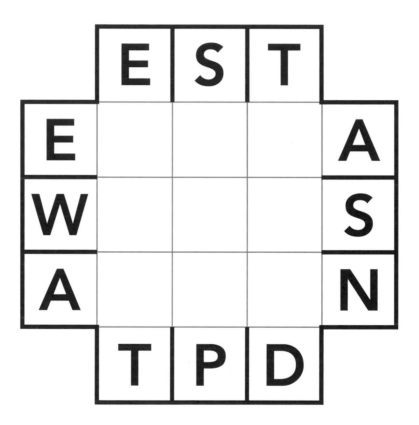

From the far east
Simply be
More than needed
Remove
Walk on
Electrical components

Maze 1

Make your way from the top of the maze to the bottom.
(Or vice versa.)

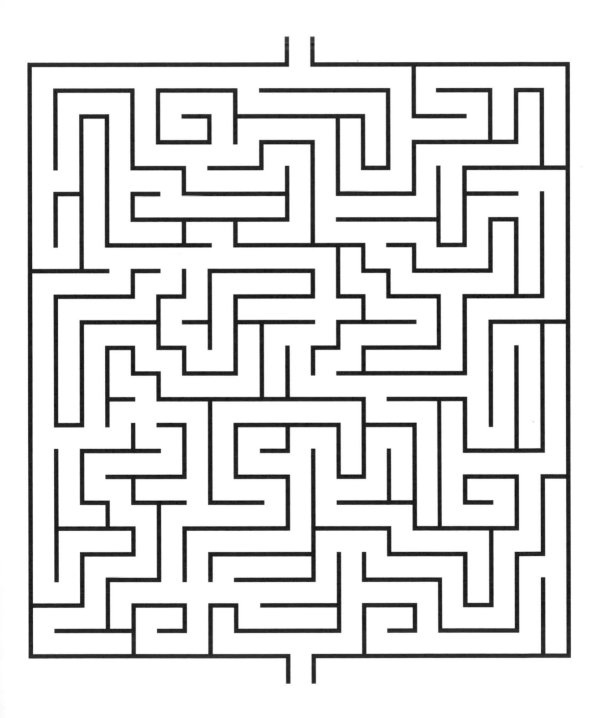

Rows Garden 2

Using the clues provided, enter a letter into each triangle to fill the garden. Each row contains one or two entries, and each hexagonal flower contains a six-letter word wrapped around the center. It's up to you to determine where to place the starting letter and the direction of the word.

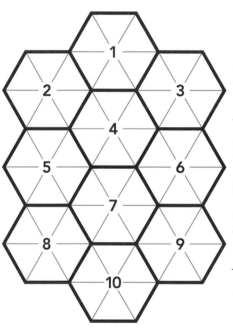

Toy Story neighbor

Pet part / Heavy metal item

Hairspray matriarch / Life-form

Ride a wave / Overflow

Green maze structure / Stationary

Mall unit / Pleased

A month / Mr. Flintstone

"Before" bit

Flowers

1.   Little landmass
2.   Hold back
3.   Still around
4.   Confound
5.   Done in haste
6.   Simple drawing
7.   Radiation counter
8.   Church leader
9.   Firefighter tool
10. Swipe

Throwing Shade 2

Shade some cells so the remaining letters in each row and column spell answers to the provided clues. Clues are sorted alphabetically by answer.

S	C	R	R	G	I	B	G	R
C	R	I	E	G	B	O	R	E
S	H	R	M	E	E	J	A	D
W	E	I	I	S	N	O	T	E
E	A	N	A	U	S	B	S	T
S	O	D	A	Y	K	R	I	E
A	R	K	C	I	R	O	B	C
T	P	O	P	S	O	Y	S	S
T	E	T	H	E	Y	R	L	R

Rows

- Curve
- Baby's bed
- A direction
- One's self
- Cosmic stuff
- One from Tulsa
- Tear apart
- Playthings
- Grape beverage

Columns

- Young man
- Task
- Stave off
- Golly!
- Pen substance
- Stretch for
- Protest
- A relative
- Perspire

Slither Fence 1

Draw a fence connecting the left and right sides of the grid along the grid lines, with no breaks, loops, or forks in the fence line. Every square with a number must be surrounded by that many fence pieces.

Transit Map 1

Use the clues to fill the bus route with letters to form words both northbound and southbound.

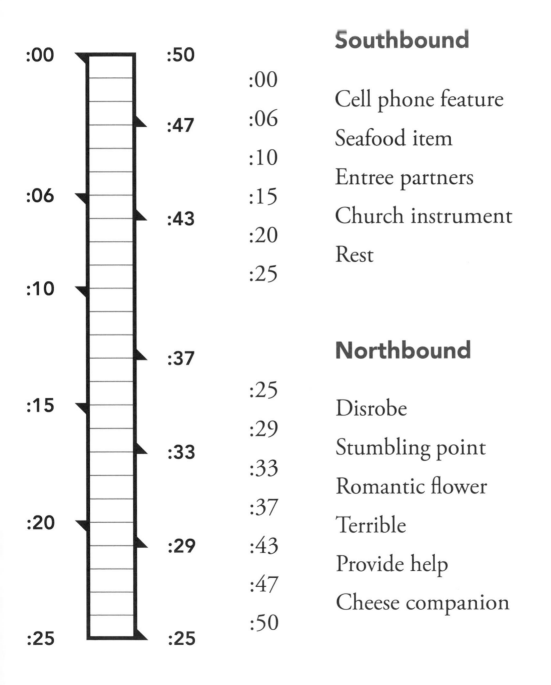

Southbound

:00 Cell phone feature

:06 Seafood item

:10 Entree partners

:15 Church instrument

:20 Rest

:25

Northbound

:25 Disrobe

:29 Stumbling point

:33 Romantic flower

:37 Terrible

:43 Provide help

:47 Cheese companion

:50

Black Holes 1

Divide the grid into chunks along the guides provided so that each chunk contains one black hole, and so the digits in the chunk sum to the number in the black hole.

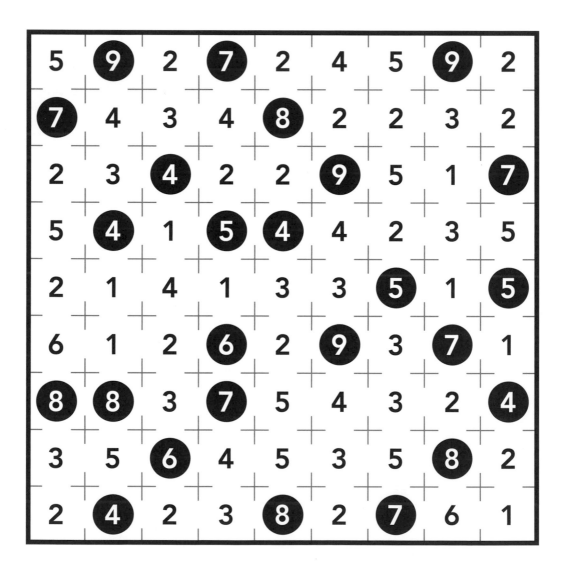

Cube Logic 3

Which of the two templates can be folded to produce the exact same block?

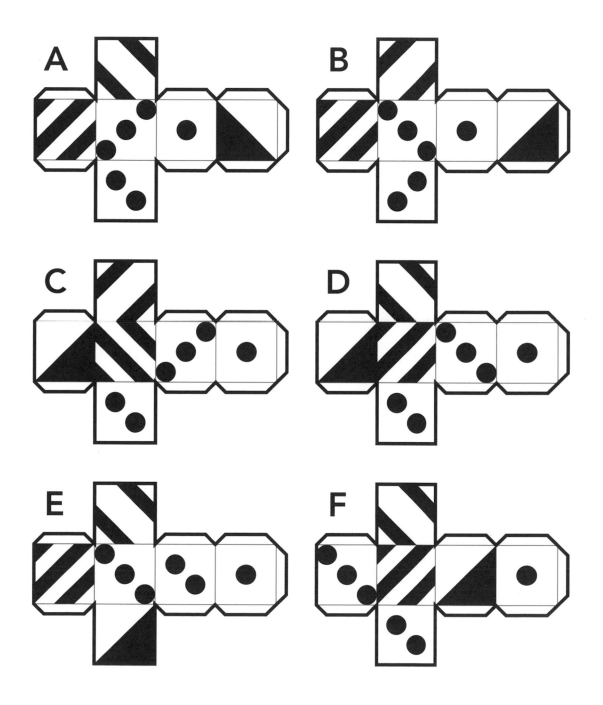

Numcross 1

Use the provided clues to fill the grid with numbers. No entry may start with a 0.

A	B	C	D		E	F
G					H	
I		■	J	K		
■		L			■	■
M	N			■	O	P
Q		■	R	S		
T		■	U			

Across

A. C down × E across

E. C down + H across

G. C down × P down

H. Sum of the digits in J across

I. A perfect cube

J. Contains only even digits

L. B down in reverse

M. R across + E down

O. I across in reverse

Q. Forms a sequence with I across and T across

R. Year the United States acquired the Virgin Islands

T. One-half of L down

U. Year Nagano hosted the winter Olympics

Down

A. I across × 6

B. A down + C down + 10

C. A perfect square

D. Digits that sum to C down

E. A palindrome

F. C down × H across

K. Another perfect square

L. T across × 2

M. K down × 3

N. Odd digits that sum to 17

O. L across − O across

P. B down + K down

S. I across + O across

NO Uncertain Terms 2

These uncertain terms have had all their letters removed except for NO. Ascertain the pairings of blanks and clues, and fill the blanks to form the answers.

N O _ _ _

_ _ N O _ N O _ _

_ N O _ _ _

_ N O _

_ _ N O _

Round feature in lumber

Type of wine

Cold being

Amateur

Pay tribute to

Finder's Fee

Can you find a number hidden within each of the sentences below? They'll add up to a nice chunk of change!

A. The fire department will use ventilators in their training program.

B. Rhonda and Kim are heading to the gym for a weightlifting session.

C. Ms. Maybel makes her famous cheesy macaroni nearly every time we have a potluck at the community center.

D. Rusty picked up a dog bone and the newspaper from the bodega.

$_ _ _ _

A B C D

Chess Sum Sudoku 2

Place a digit from 1 to 5 into each empty cell so that each row, column, and 2 × 3 block contains each digit once, without repetition. The chess knights in the grid display the sum of the digits in the cells which they can attack.

Transit Map 2

Use the clues to fill the bus route with letters to form words both northbound and southbound.

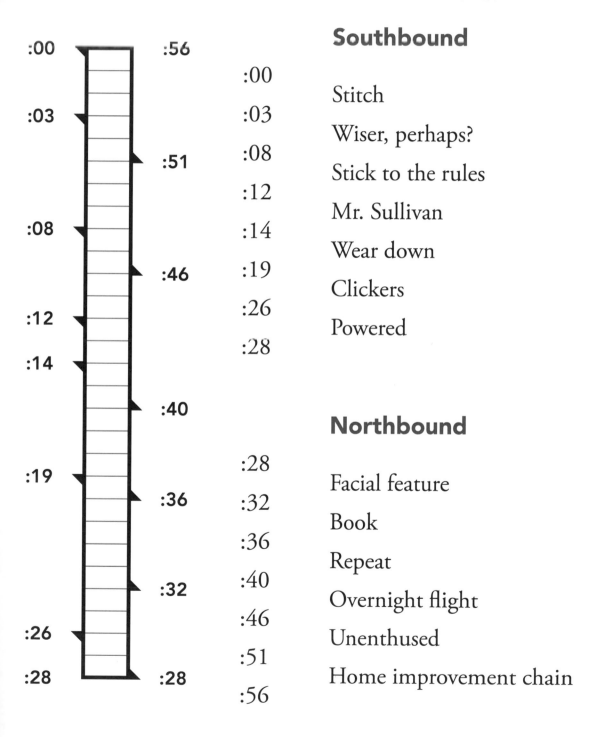

Southbound

:00 Stitch

:03 Wiser, perhaps?

:08 Stick to the rules

:12 Mr. Sullivan

:14 Wear down

:19 Clickers

:26 Powered

:28

Northbound

:28 Facial feature

:32 Book

:36 Repeat

:40 Overnight flight

:46 Unenthused

:51 Home improvement chain

:56

Rows Garden 3

Using the clues provided, enter a letter into each triangle to fill the garden. Each row contains one or two entries, and each hexagonal flower contains a six-letter word wrapped around the center. It's up to you to determine where to place the starting letter and the direction of the word.

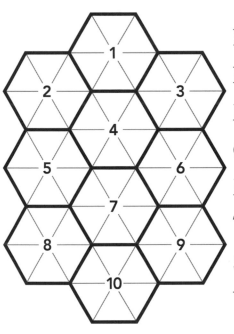

Himalayan tea

Leader / Map line type

Memo / Powerless

Chop / Celebrity

Mix / Shoot!

Take a spin / A symptom

Started / Classify

VCR opt.

Flowers

1. Some seats
2. An east coast US city
3. Change back
4. Some younger ladies
5. Swift and precise
6. Sauce served with fish
7. Protect
8. Span
9. Noah of *The Daily Show*
10. Solution

Sudoku TV 2

Place one of each letter from MATLOCK into each row, column, and boldly outlined region.

T			K	M		
					L	
M	A	T	L	O	C	K
	M					
		L	C			T

Word Funnel 2

Fill each section of the funnel with a six-letter word made up of the six letters above it. Clues have been provided in no particular order.

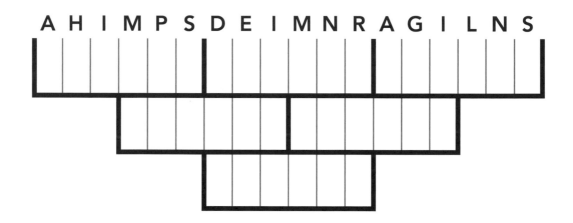

Eight-legged creature

Building material

Little accident

Help someone who forgot

Space for dirty clothing

An alert or notice

Woven Words 3

Use the clues to weave six words together in the grid below; three going across and three going down. The unwoven letters have been placed to get you started.

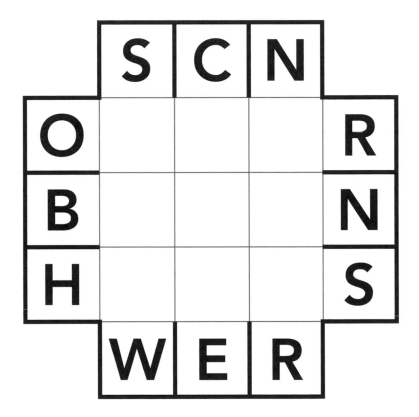

Common dirt color

Task

Tortoise foes

More recent

None of the above

Farm material

Cube Logic 4

Which of the four foldable patterns can be folded to make the block displayed?

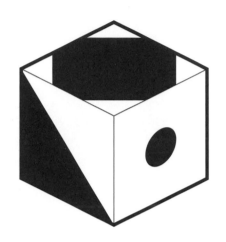

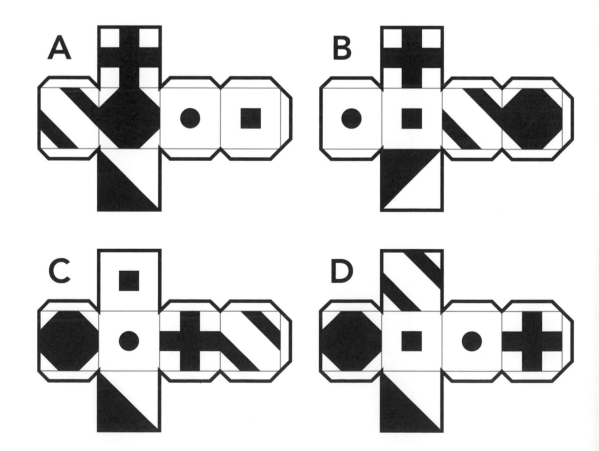

Rearrangement 3 & 4

Rearrange the letters in TOFU OBLONGS to spell somewhere you might find faux meat as an ingredient.

Rearrange the letters in A DAILY TROPHY to spell an event where the best ugly sweater is likely to win awards.

Black Holes 2

Divide the grid into chunks along the guides provided so that each chunk contains one black hole, and so the digits in the chunk sum to the number in the black hole.

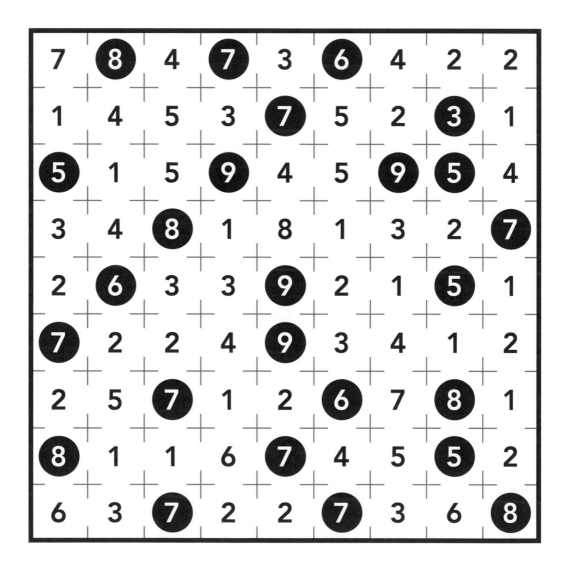

Transit Map 3

Use the clues to fill the bus route with letters to form words both northbound and southbound.

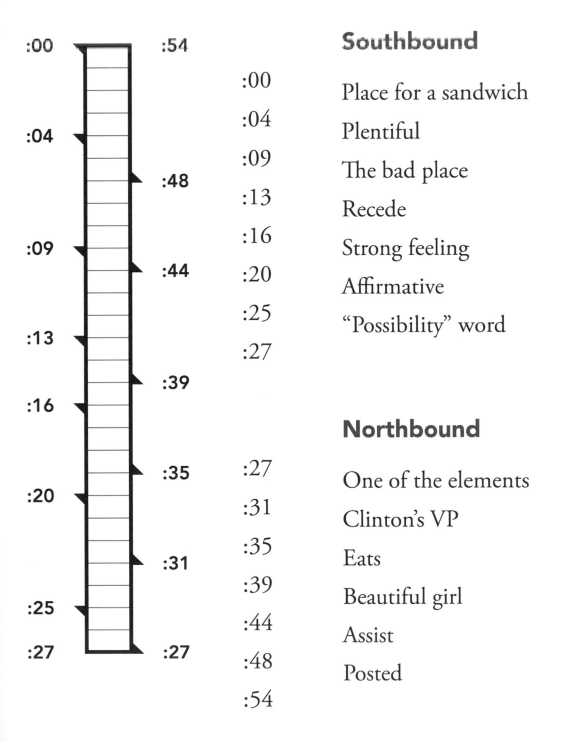

:00   :54

:04

            :48

:09

            :44

:13

            :39

:16

            :35

:20

            :31

:25

:27   :27

Southbound

:00   Place for a sandwich

:04   Plentiful

:09   The bad place

:13   Recede

:16   Strong feeling

:20   Affirmative

:25   "Possibility" word

:27

Northbound

:27   One of the elements

:31   Clinton's VP

:35   Eats

:39   Beautiful girl

:44   Assist

:48   Posted

:54

Throwing Shade 3

Shade some cells so the remaining letters in each row and column spell answers to the provided clues. Clues are sorted alphabetically by answer.

C	G	A	N	T	E	W	T	S
L	S	A	V	U	R	G	T	E
A	A	N	I	N	S	O	E	R
L	O	F	V	I	E	N	D	E
E	O	C	A	T	S	O	L	A
N	S	H	H	E	A	S	U	L
A	N	T	I	I	L	S	E	D
S	G	O	L	L	D	E	N	A
P	E	R	E	S	R	E	S	S

Rows

- Stellar spice
- Some pets
- A fizzy drink
- Bright and shiny
- Recover
- Deep attraction
- A simple answer
- The media
- Sudden rush

Columns

- Item on a ship
- Applaud
- Duck follower
- Camera part
- Use a book
- Enclosure
- Musical performance
- Day before Wed.
- Repugnant

Penny Candy 2

Penny candy has gone up in price a fair bit. Use the total prices of the sets of four candies to figure out how much each piece of candy costs.

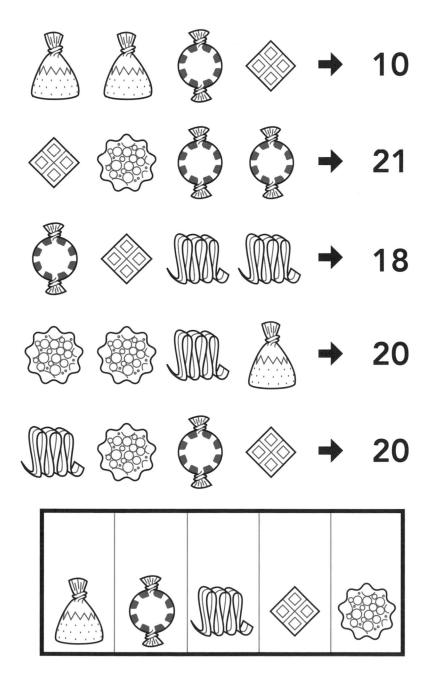

Word Funnel 3

Fill each section of the funnel with a six-letter word made up of the six letters above it. Clues have been provided in no particular order.

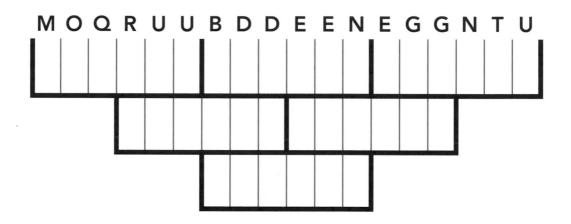

M O Q R U U B D D E E N E G G N T U

Curved and misaligned

Piece of chicken

Phone user's information

Minimum viable group of people

Weight to bear

Moved slightly

Rearrangement 5 & 6

Rearrange the letters in PORCH PLAN + ANKLE to spell a way you might ruffle some feathers besides ringing a doorbell and running away.

Rearrange the letters in ARRANGES SHED to spell an item you might find out in the shed.

Numcross 2

Use the provided clues to fill the grid with numbers.
No entry may start with a 0.

A	B	C			D	E
F			G		H	
		I		J		
	K			L		
M			N			
O			P		Q	R
S				T		

Across

A. One-half of M down

D. R down in reverse

F. D down in reverse

H. One-third of R down

I. Contains one of every even digit

K. A perfect cube

L. D across – 2

M. I across × 3

O. D across + H across

P. One-twentieth of I across

S. Q down × 2

T. Digits that sum to H across

Down

A. R down – 5

B. S across + 2

C. A multiple of O across

D. Two pair

E. G down × 5

G. Another perfect cube

J. I across scrambled

K. Digits that sum to 15

M. A across × 2

N. A perfect square

Q. One-half of S across

R. Another perfect square

Woven Words 4

Use the clues to weave six words together in the grid below; three going across and three going down. The unwoven letters have been placed to get you started.

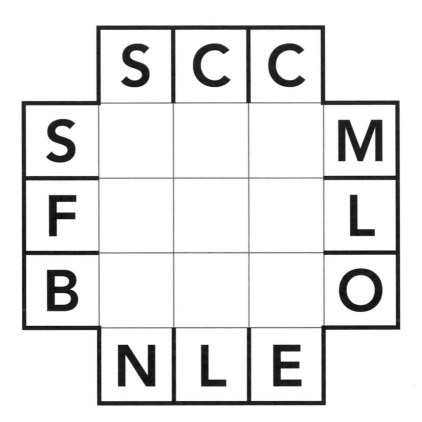

A word of applause

Pinkish color

Have an intense desire

Wild like some cats

Severe

Some rough weather

Rows Garden 4

Using the clues provided, enter a letter into each triangle to fill the garden. Each row contains one or two entries, and each hexagonal flower contains a six-letter word wrapped around the center. It's up to you to determine where to place the starting letter and the direction of the word.

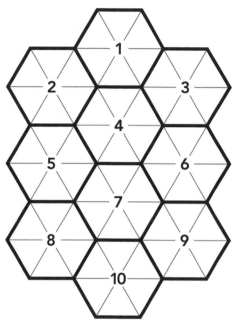

Diminished

Feature of a corner / Quit

Giveaway / Elegant bird

Type of plant / Toxic substance

Pointy shape / Row in a store

Belief system / Mythos

Common size / Wealthy

A card

Flowers

1. Comrade
2. Make a mess of
3. Borrowed
4. Witty
5. Goodies
6. Optimist's fruits
7. Get off track
8. Beats together
9. Brave, courageous
10. Take back

Transit Map 4

Use the clues to fill the bus route with letters to form words both northbound and southbound.

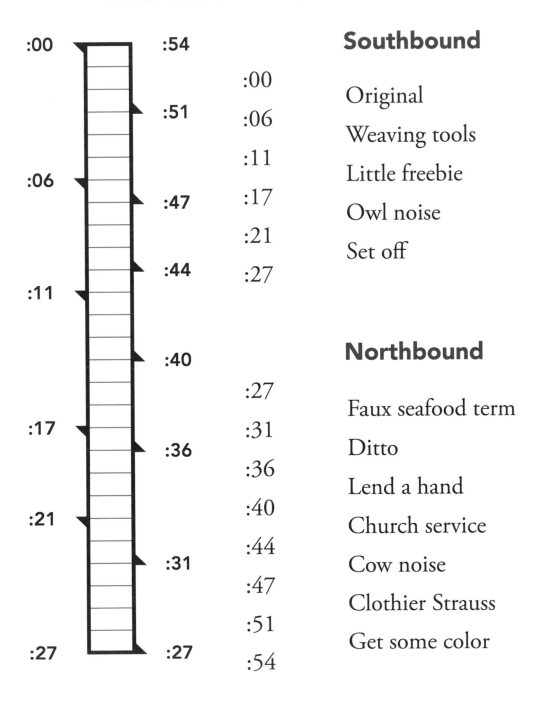

Southbound

:00 Original

:06 Weaving tools

:11 Little freebie

:17 Owl noise

:21 Set off

:27

Northbound

:27 Faux seafood term

:31 Ditto

:36 Lend a hand

:40 Church service

:44 Cow noise

:47 Clothier Strauss

:51 Get some color

:54

Maze 2

Make your way from the top of the maze to the bottom.
(Or vice versa.)

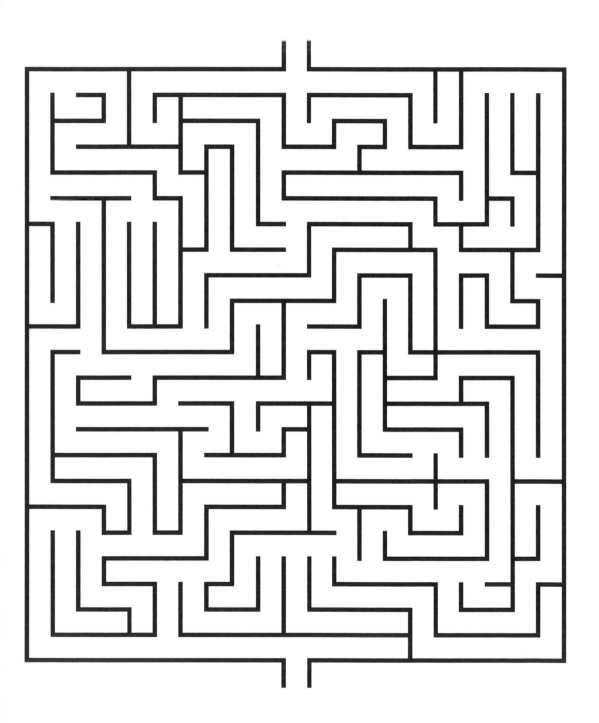

Slither Fence 2

Draw a fence connecting the left and right sides of the grid along the grid lines, with no breaks, loops, or forks in the fence line. Every square with a number must be surrounded by that many fence pieces.

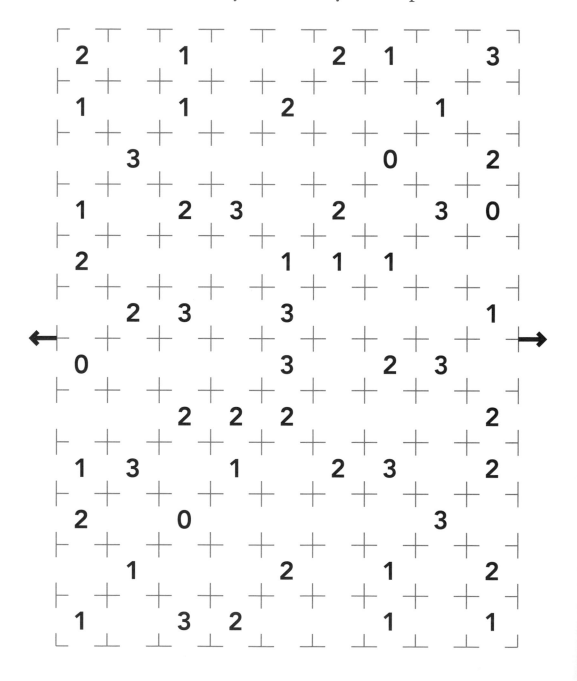

Word Funnel 4

Fill each section of the funnel with a six-letter word made up of the six letters above it. Clues have been provided in no particular order.

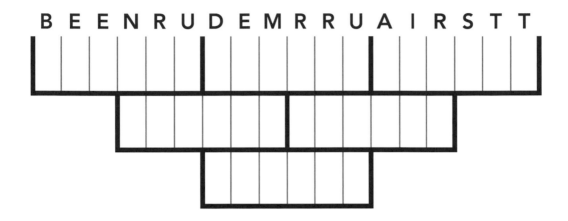

B E E N R U D E M R R U A I R S T T

One who paints or sculpts
One who works on Wall Street
One way to exchange goods
One possible crime drama topic
One type of sandwich
One, e.g.

Black Holes 3

Divide the grid into chunks along the guides provided so that each chunk contains one black hole, and so the digits in the chunk sum to the number in the black hole.

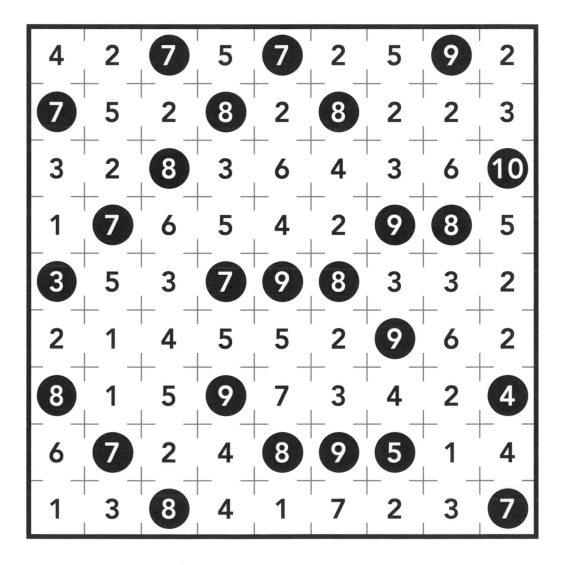

Throwing Shade 4

Shade some cells so the remaining letters in each row and column spell answers to the provided clues. Clues are sorted alphabetically by answer.

M	K	E	C	S	T	T	T	S
O	R	A	R	S	I	E	S	T
G	K	N	I	T	E	W	E	S
S	T	E	U	N	O	T	A	T
E	W	A	M	U	N	A	R	T
O	E	G	O	B	E	G	U	O
S	E	G	T	A	E	N	T	O
W	Y	E	B	A	R	N	T	N
D	Y	R	A	R	R	E	N	E

Rows

- Headpiece
- Self
- Flying things
- Became acquainted with
- Rest area
- Steak preference
- Athlete info
- Reporter's pad
- Desire

Columns

- Ready and willing
- Tiny bit
- Type of lime
- Sea parter
- Heat briskly
- Gas ball
- Rock
- Light brown
- Level

Cube Logic 5

Which of the four foldable patterns can be folded to make the block displayed?

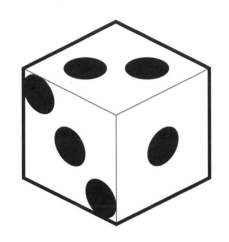

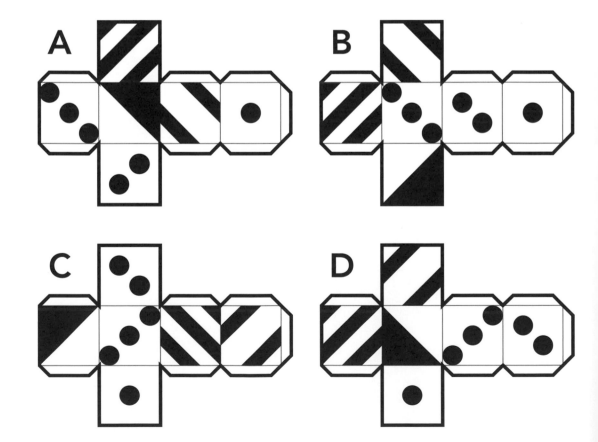

Chess Sum Sudoku 3

Place a digit from 1 to 8 into each empty cell so that each row, column, and 3 × 3 block contains each digit once, without repetition. The chess knights in the grid display the sum of the digits in the cells which they can attack.

Numcross 3

Use the provided clues to fill the grid with numbers. No entry may start with a 0.

A	B	C	D		E	F
G					H	
I			J	K		
		L				
M	N				O	P
Q			R	S		
T			U			

Across

A. A palindrome

E. Digits that sum to T across

G. Some combination of digits from M down and O across

H. B down – M down

I. Square root of M down

J. A down × Q across

L. One-half of N down

M. B down × 7

O. One-fifth of H across

Q. A perfect square

R. Consecutive digits, not in order

T. Forms a sequence with O across and C down

U. Consecutive digits in ascending order

Down

A. B down + 100

B. M down + H across

C. I across × 2

D. A palindrome

E. P down + 1

F. M down × 5

K. I across × 7

L. A perfect cube

M. I across squared

N. Another palindrome

O. Q across × 7

P. S down × T across

S. Another perfect square

Transit Map 5

Use the clues to fill the bus route with letters to form words both northbound and southbound.

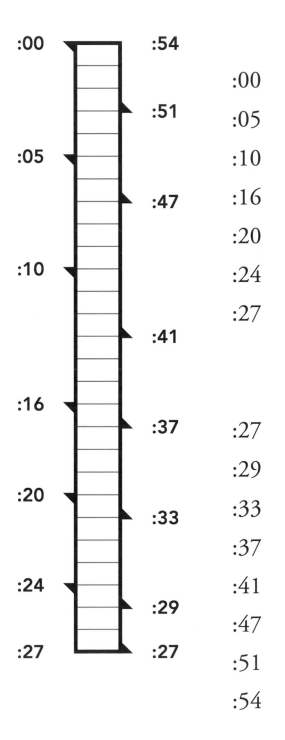

Southbound

Quick breakfast

State

Small airplane brand

Cast a ballot

Flying toy

A tuber

Northbound

Pa's wife

Abominable snowman

No-carb diet

Skater shoe brand

Covert

Dancer's garb

Sign of agreement

Woven Words 5

Use the clues to weave six words together in the grid below;
three going across and three going down. The unwoven
letters have been placed to get you started.

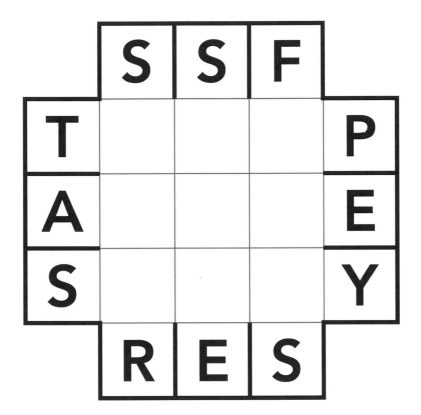

Nimble

Theater offerings

Entertainer Davis Jr.

Ooze

A baking ingredient

A flower

Black Holes 4

Divide the grid into chunks along the guides provided so that each chunk contains one black hole, and so the digits in the chunk sum to the number in the black hole.

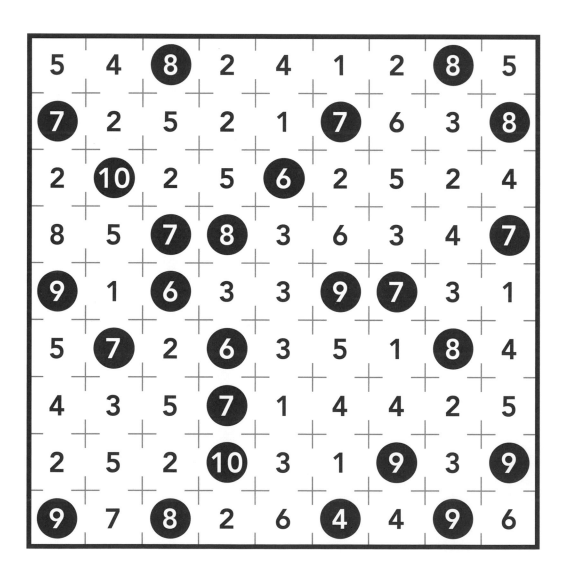

Rearrangement 7 & 8

Rearrange the letters in GLARING GOOD to spell a forest path where a good line of sight is always welcome.

Rearrange the letters in CYBORG GEAR to spell something that's more useful to a human that runs on food than a robot that runs on electricity.

Penny Candy 3

Penny candy has gone up in price a fair bit. Use the total prices of the sets of four candies to figure out how much each piece of candy costs.

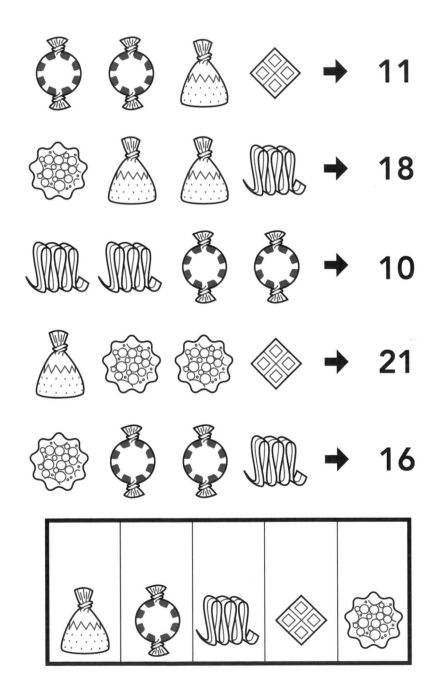

Word Funnel 5

Fill each section of the funnel with a six-letter word made up of the six letters above it. Clues have been provided in no particular order.

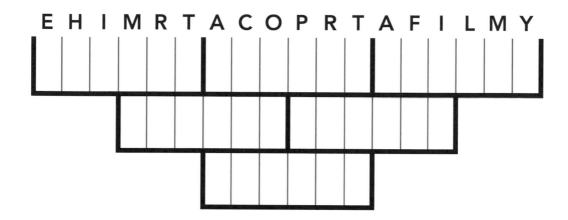

E H I M R T A C O P R T A F I L M Y

Affect

One's kin

A dedicated loner

Consideration

A known arrangement or setup

A chess player, at times

Transit Map 6

Use the clues to fill the bus route with letters to form words both northbound and southbound.

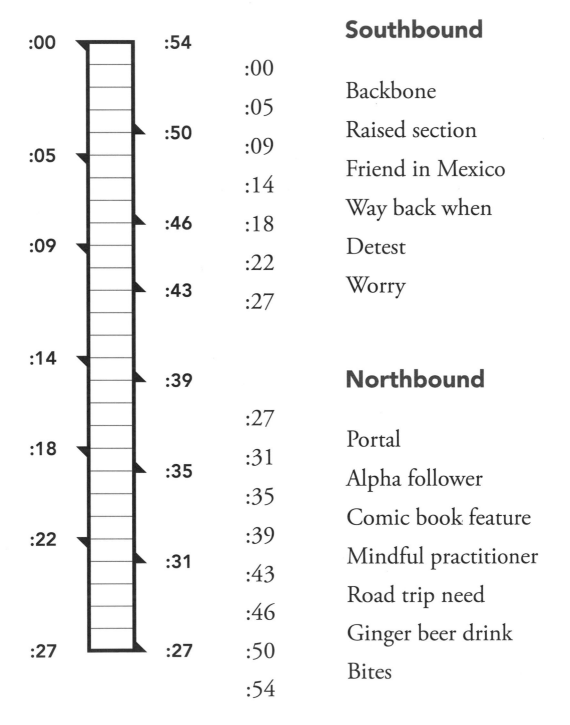

Southbound

:00
:05 Backbone
:09 Raised section
:14 Friend in Mexico
:18 Way back when
:22 Detest
:27 Worry

Northbound

:27
:31 Portal
:35 Alpha follower
:39 Comic book feature
:43 Mindful practitioner
:46 Road trip need
:50 Ginger beer drink
:54 Bites

Sudoku TV 3

Place one of each letter from DRAGNET into each row, column, and boldly outlined region.

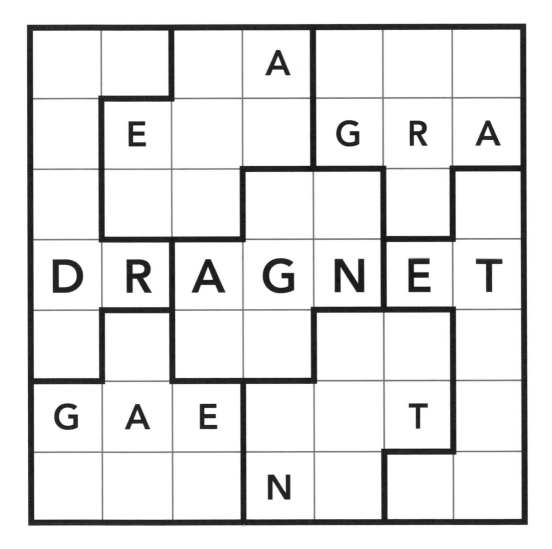

Cube Logic 6

Which of the four foldable patterns can be folded to make the block displayed?

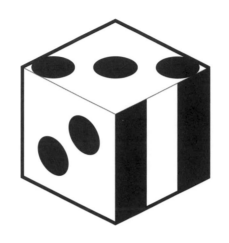

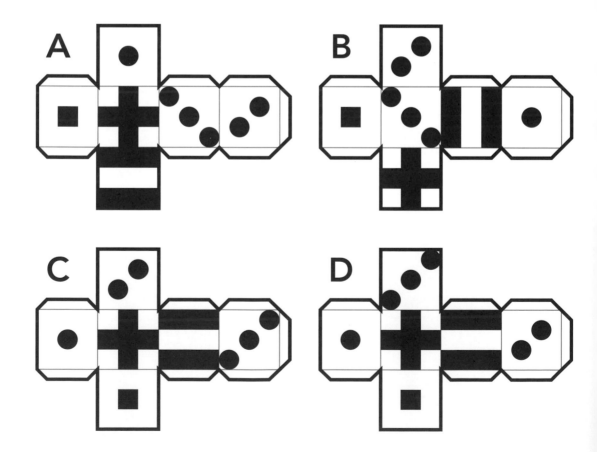

Throwing Shade 5

Shade some cells so the remaining letters in each row and column spell answers to the provided clues. Clues are sorted alphabetically by answer.

T	T	U	B	E	B	F	E	T
K	I	S	C	W	A	R	I	F
P	T	E	A	X	C	H	X	I
A	A	B	L	B	L	E	L	F
T	L	O	K	I	A	W	I	I
L	I	S	S	N	S	L	T	N
M	N	M	E	T	R	I	C	L
C	C	O	E	O	S	N	T	E
C	T	O	A	D	A	D	N	D

Rows

- Can-do
- Ice cream holder
- Fuzzy fruit
- Something of Santa's
- Man on the moon
- Cold-weather gear
- Yellow cab
- An amphibian
- System used in London?

Columns

- Lightweight wood
- Related to life
- Baked good
- Way out
- Grind down
- VHS courtesy
- Type of powder
- Color
- Bob Hope org.

Chess Sum Sudoku 4

Place a digit from 1 to 8 into each empty cell so that each row, column, and 3 × 3 block contains each digit once, without repetition. The chess knights in the grid display the sum of the digits in the cells which they can attack.

NO Uncertain Terms 3

These uncertain terms have had all their letters removed except for NO. Ascertain the pairings of blanks and clues, and fill the blanks to form the answers.

_ _ N O _ _ _ _ _

N O _ _ _ _

_ _ _ _ _ N O

_ N O _ _ _ _ _ _

_ _ N O _ _ _ _

Lennon's wife

Information

Boy with a growing nose

Refurbish

Document signing witness

Numcross 4

Use the provided clues to fill the grid with numbers. No entry may start with a 0.

Across

A. Forms a sequence with T down and V across

C. S down squared

F. H across in reverse

H. A perfect square

I. One-half of B down

K. C down + S down

L. Contains one of each even digit

N. T down – 1

O. Another perfect square

P. Digits that sum to 20

R. U across + 100

U. M down + N across

V. Another perfect square

Down

A. B down – 10

B. A perfect cube

C. A pair

D. Contains every non-zero even digit

E. H across + 800

G. A multiple of S down

J. C down × K across

L. One-eighth of L across

M. Q down × T down

N. N across × S down

Q. S down in reverse

S. The square root of C across

T. Sum of the digits in L down

Rows Garden 5

Using the clues provided, enter a letter into each triangle to fill the garden. Each row contains one or two entries, and each hexagonal flower contains a six-letter word wrapped around the center. It's up to you to determine where to place the starting letter and the direction of the word.

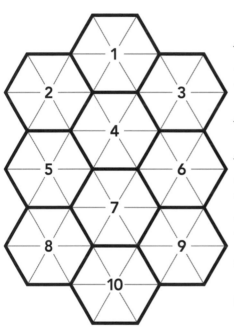

A vehicle

Put on TV / Speak

A country in S.A. / 37th US President

A month

Metropolis / Shred

Delicate wood / Terrible

Old item / Regal one

Common phone co. suffix

Flowers

1. Followed a path
2. Fix
3. Noise maker
4. Tiny
5. Waste system
6. Type of discount
7. Oily and slick
8. Sports player?
9. Still kickin'
10. Graze lightly

Woven Words 6

Use the clues to weave six words together in the grid below; three going across and three going down. Unlike earlier puzzles of this type, the unwoven letters are provided but not placed.

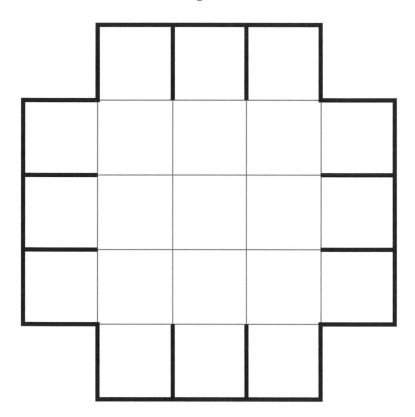

AAEEMNOPRRST

Around

By oneself

One of your pearly whites

Tex-Mex bean

Batman's buddy

Cook in oil

Numcross 5

Use the provided clues to fill the grid with numbers. No entry may start with a 0.

A	B	C		D	E	F
G				H		
		I	J		K	
	L			M		
N			O			
P		Q		R	S	T
U				V		

Across

A. D across in reverse

D. U across × 3

G. A palindrome

H. G across + 1

I. A perfect cube

K. Q down + 4

L. A "full house"

N. A down – B down

O. I across + 5

P. A down + N down

R. Another palindrome

U. T down × 5

V. L across / Q down

Down

A. One-half of H across

B. N across – D down

C. D down × H across

D. K across + 2

E. N across × Q down

F. A across + 16

J. Consecutive digits in ascending order

L. A multiple of T down

M. G across × K across

N. N across × 11

Q. A perfect square

S. Q down × 2

T. Q down – 4

Black Holes 5

Divide the grid into chunks along the guides provided so that each chunk contains one black hole, and so the digits in the chunk sum to the number in the black hole.

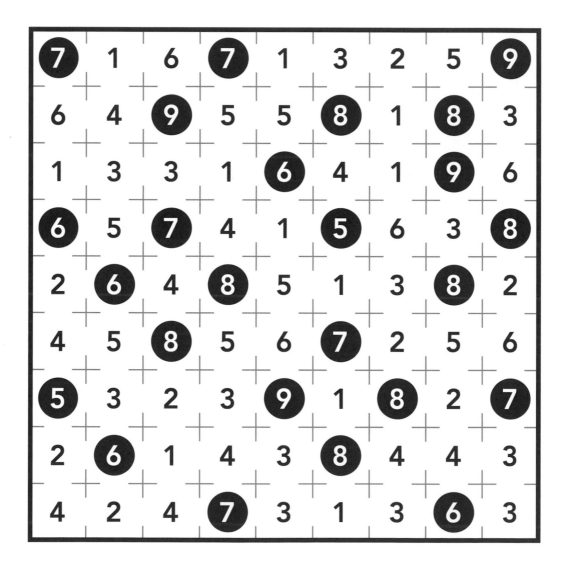

Word Funnel 6

Fill each section of the funnel with a six-letter word made up of the six letters above it. Clues have been provided in no particular order.

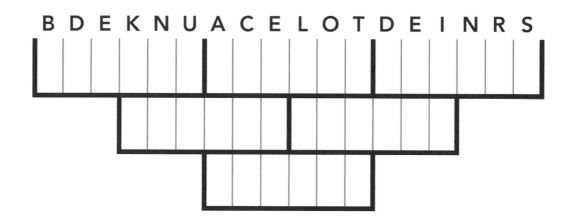

Washed off

Dispel disinformation

Vessel used by NASA

To find

Keep

Open

Cube Logic 7

Which of the four foldable patterns can be folded to make the block displayed?

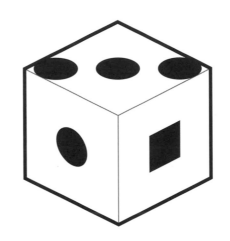

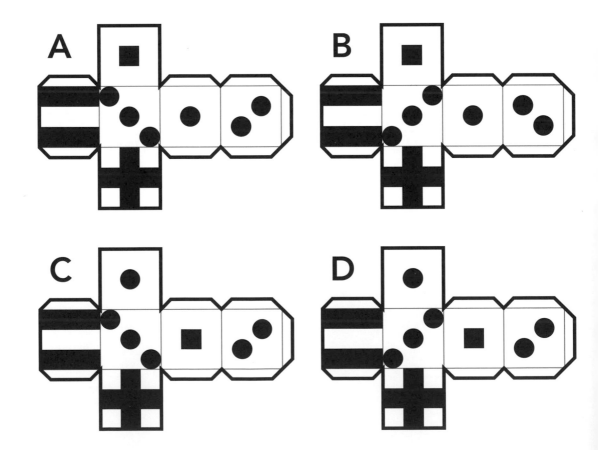

A

B

C

D

Slither Fence 3

Draw a fence connecting the left and right sides of the grid along the grid lines, with no breaks, loops, or forks in the fence line. Every square with a number must be surrounded by that many fence pieces.

Numcross 6

Use the provided clues to fill the grid with numbers. No entry may start with a 0.

A	B	C		D	E	F
G				H		
		I	J		K	
	L			M		
N			O			
P		Q		R	S	T
U				V		

Across

A. A down + F down

D. A down × D down

G. F down + 19

H. F down scrambled

I. A perfect square

K. B down – O across

L. Contains one of every even digit

N. A down – 1

O. A perfect cube

P. Consecutive digits in descending order

R. Digits that sum to 16

U. D across × 2

V. A palindrome

Down

A. D down – 20

B. A down × 7

C. Year George H. W. Bush was first elected US President

D. O across + 4

E. I across × K across

F. L across / G across

J. O across × 6

L. C down + K across

M. Another palindrome

N. H across + S down

Q. A down × 2

S. A multiple of N across

T. O across × 2

Sudoku TV 4

Place one of each unique letter from DICK VAN DYKE into each row, column, and 3 × 3 block.

			C			E		V
					Y		I	
D	I	C	K					A
							V	
K			V	A	N			Y
	E							
I					D	Y	K	E
	C		A					
Y		D		V				

Transit Map 7

Use the clues to fill the bus route with letters to form words both northbound and southbound.

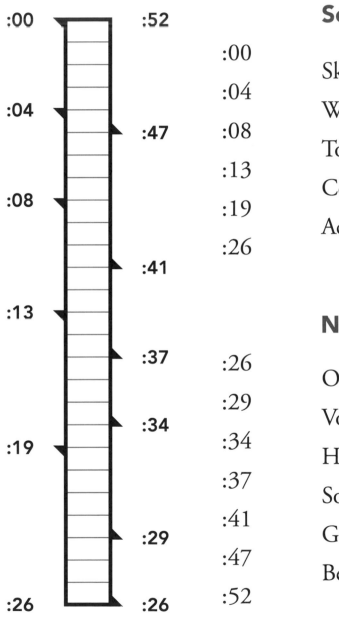

Southbound

:00 Skin problem

:04 Whirl

:08 Tortilla constructs

:13 Collide

:19 Actress Holm

:26

Northbound

:26 Off-planet beings

:29 Vote into office

:34 Hat

:37 Soybean paste

:41 Greens for kitties

:47 Beverage mover

:52

Chess Sum Sudoku 5

Place a digit from 1 to 8 into each empty cell so that each row, column, and 3 × 3 block contains each digit once, without repetition. The chess knights in the grid display the sum of the digits in the cells which they can attack.

Woven Words 7

Use the clues to weave six words together in the grid below; three going across and three going down. Unlike earlier puzzles of this type, the unwoven letters are provided but not placed.

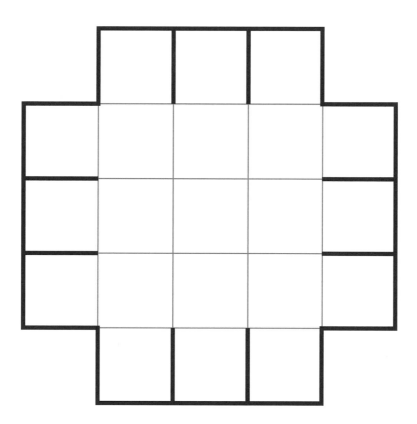

ABCDEGLRSSTY

Type of fruit

Mean-spirited

Underwater worker

Group of trees

Brownish tone

Kettle part

Penny Candy 4

Penny candy has gone up in price a fair bit. Use the total prices of the sets of four candies to figure out how much each piece of candy costs.

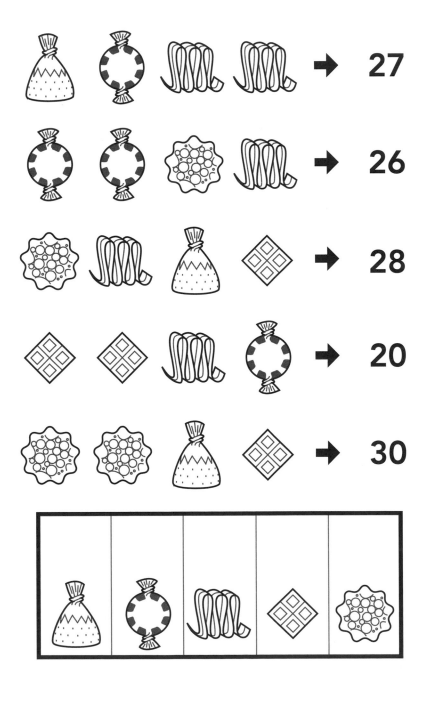

Maze 3

Make your way from the top of the maze to the bottom.
(Or vice versa.)

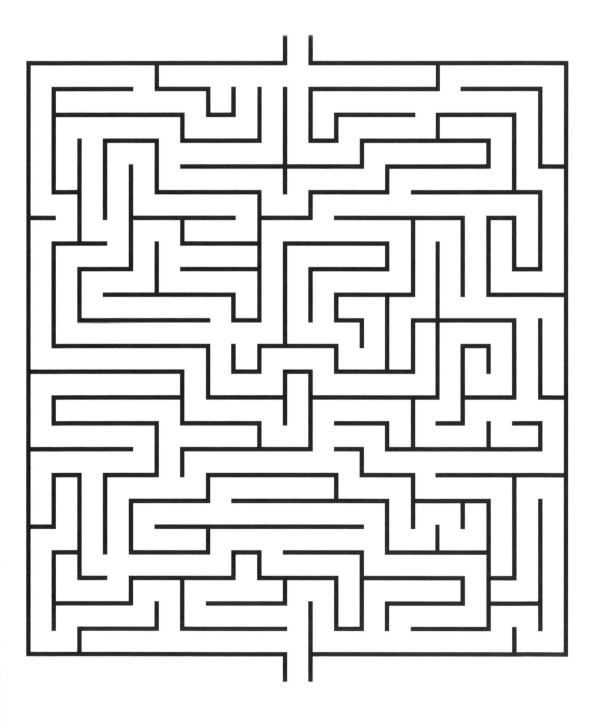

Numcross 7

Use the provided clues to fill the grid with numbers. No entry may start with a 0.

A	B		C	D	E		F	G
H			I				J	
K		L			M	N		
O				P				
		Q	R			S	T	U
V	W		X		Y		Z	
AA		BB		CC		DD		
		EE	FF			GG	HH	II
JJ	KK				LL			
MM			NN	OO			PP	
QQ			RR				SS	

Across

A. Sum of the digits in K across

C. AA across scrambled

F. DD down / J across

H. QQ across – V down

I. Z across × J across

J. Square root of N down

K. KK down × J across

M. K across + H across

O. A palindrome that's one-fifth of LL across

P. N down × 2

Q. One-fifth of NN across

S. W down × 2

V. V down + 3

X. Another palindrome

Z. OO down – 10

AA. A perfect cube

CC. U down × Z across

EE. Consecutive digits in descending order

GG. W down × J across

JJ. Comprised of digits under 5

LL. FF down in reverse

MM. Digits that sum to J across

NN. Q across × 5

PP. J across + 2

QQ. H across + V down

RR. LL down + 10

SS. A perfect square

Down

A. Consecutive digits, not in order

B. Year the Seahawks first won the Super Bowl

C. C across + H across

D. Another perfect square

E. M across scrambled

F. RR across – 5

G. JJ down × 5

(Continued)

L. J across × U down

N. Another palindrome

P. Contains one of every even digit

R. T down – 5

T. Another perfect cube

U. D down – 4

V. OO down in reverse

W. Another perfect square

Y. NN across – EE across

BB. PP across × H across

DD. S across + D down

FF. One-fourth of P down

HH. Digits that sum to A across

II. AA across × 3

JJ. PP across × J across

KK. One-half of NN across

LL. One-sixth of EE across

OO. V down in reverse

Cube Logic 8

Which of the four foldable patterns can be folded to make the block displayed?

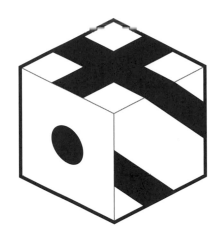

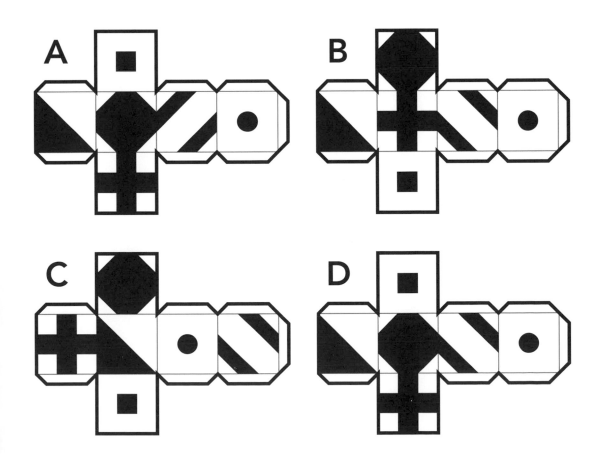

A

B

C

D

Word Funnel 7

Fill each section of the funnel with a six-letter word made up of the six letters above it. Clues have been provided in no particular order.

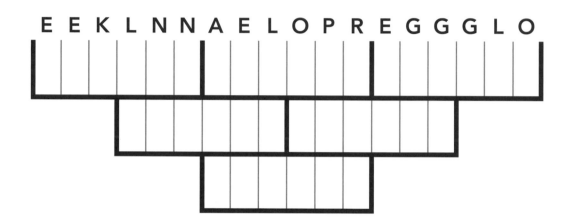

E E K L N N A E L O P R E G G G L O

Place for an animal

Big name in web searches

A woodworking tool

Prisoner's goal

A state in the Pacific Northwest

Stare in disbelief

Sudoku TV 5

Place one of each unique letter from BRADY BUNCH into each row, column, and 3 × 3 block.

D		H		C				U
			Y		H		B	
B	R			N		A		
		A	D	Y				
U								B
			B	U	N			
		R		U			C	H
	C		A		B			
N				D		U		Y

Numcross 8

Use the provided clues to fill the grid with numbers. No entry may start with a 0.

A	B	C		D	E		F	G
H				I			J	
		K	L		M	N		
	O			P		Q		
R				S	T			
U			V				W	X
		Y					Z	
	AA			BB	CC	DD		
EE			FF		GG			
HH			II	JJ		KK	LL	MM
NN			OO			PP		

Across

A. Y across in reverse

D. D down – 1

F. One-half of R down

H. A perfect square

I. B down + D down

J. X down – 6

K. One-tenth of S across

M. Digits that sum to LL down

O. Year the US Congress passed the 22nd Amendment

Q. F across × 3

R. AA across × 5

S. H across × 5

U. A perfect cube

V. Three of a kind

W. Another perfect square

Y. V across + V down

Z. F across – 5

AA. S across / R across

BB. Two pair

EE. AA down scrambled

GG. F across × 3

HH. A multiple of L down

II. JJ down – Z across

KK. R down × 7

NN. A down + 7

OO. One-half of LL down

PP. S across – X down

Down

A. B down + U across

B. Another perfect cube

C. One-fifth of P down

D. Sum of the digits in E down

E. PP across + L down

F. F across × G down

G. One-eighth of W down

L. Another perfect square

N. A multiple of LL down

O. A down + X down

(Continued)

P.   Contains one of every odd digit

R.   R across + 2

T.   Sum of the digits in C down

V.   Another perfect square

W.   G down × 8

X.   Another perfect square

Y.   O down × 3

AA.   A multiple of E down

CC.   Another perfect square

DD.   BB across – O down

EE.   Consecutive digits, not in order

FF.   EE across / OO across

JJ.   Z across + II across

LL.   Sum of the digits in M across

MM.   A pair

Woven Words 8

Use the clues to weave six words together in the grid below; three going across and three going down. Unlike earlier puzzles of this type, the unwoven letters are provided but not placed.

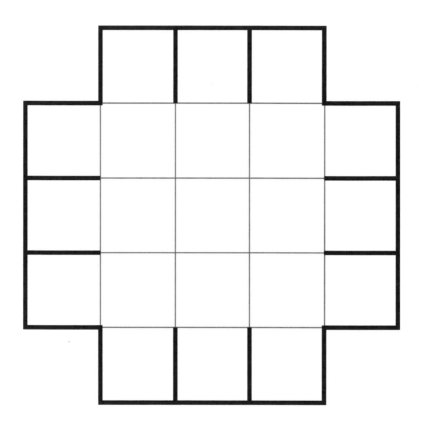

CCDEGHILRSTY

Something in space

Offense

Croc cousin

Robust

Kept running in place

Motionless

NO Uncertain Terms 4

These uncertain terms have had all their letters removed
except for NO. Ascertain the pairings of blanks and clues,
and fill the blanks to form the answers.

_ _ _ _ _ N O

_ _ N O _ _ _ _

N O _ _ _ _ _ _ _

N O _ _ _ _

_ N O _

Flooring material option
Pretentious jerk
A country in Scandinavia
Lava-producing feature
Where you'd find Oregon and Washington

Cube Logic 9

Which of the four foldable patterns can be folded to make the block displayed?

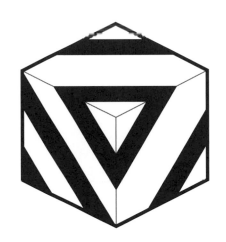

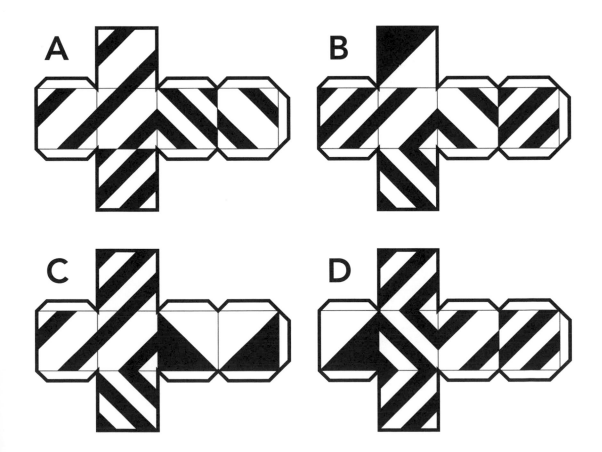

Numcross 9

Use the provided clues to fill the grid with numbers. No entry may start with a 0.

A	B		C	D	E		F	G
H			I				J	
K		L			M	N		
O				P				
		Q	R			S	T	U
V	W		X		Y		Z	
AA		BB		CC		DD		
		EE	FF			GG	HH	II
JJ	KK				LL			
MM			NN	OO			PP	
QQ			RR				SS	

Across

A. D down – 1

C. A palindrome

F. H across + 4

H. A across in reverse

I. D down × 2

J. Number of ones in the top three rows of the puzzle

K. Four of a kind

M. P down / Z across

O. A multiple of J across

P. I across × 2

Q. J across squared

S. A perfect cube

V. R down in reverse

X. J across × V across

Z. One-third of D down

AA. LL down × 3

CC. An anagram of C across

EE. Y down × MM across

GG. CC across – 100

JJ. N down × 9

LL. HH down + T down

MM. One-fifth of D down

NN. RR across – J across

PP. F across + SS across

QQ. H across + SS across

RR. J across × PP across

SS. E down / LL down

Down

A. The digits of H across and PP across scrambled

B. Digits that sum to MM across

C. LL down + SS across

D. Number of unshaded squares in the grid

E. K across – LL down

F. H across × J across

G. P across – L down

L. Another palindrome

N. OO down × 3

(Continued)

P. Contains one of each odd digit

R. Another perfect cube

T. J across × 2

U. J across × 5

V. V across + 1

W. SS across × 2

Y. One-eighth of DD down

BB. AA across + R down

DD. M across – K across

FF. Year the last new episode of *The Dick Van Dyke Show* first aired

HH. Year President Abraham Lincoln took office

II. E down + P across

JJ. C down + 4

KK. Digits that sum to W down

LL. K across / J across

OO. QQ across + SS across

Transit Map 8

Use the clues to fill the bus route with letters to form words both northbound and southbound.

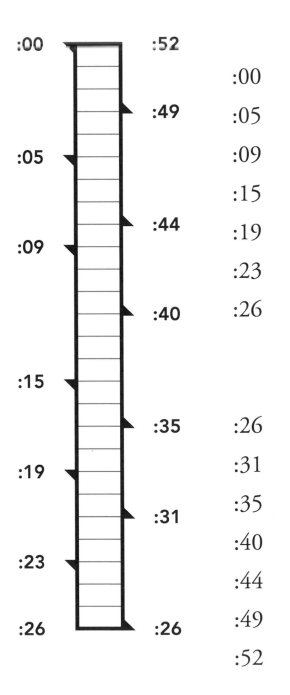

:00   :52

:49

:05

:44

:09

:40

:15

:35

:19

:31

:23

:26   :26

Southbound

:00

:05 Road trip stop

:09 Shoot

:15 Type of verse

:19 Metal wrap

:23 Ones or elevens

:26 Hip-hop

Northbound

:26

:31 Decipher

:35 Pac. Coast state

:40 Routinely

:44 Front of a plane

:49 Hunter's tool

:52 Mr. Hanks or Cruise

Woven Words 9

Use the clues to weave six words together in the grid below; three going across and three going down. Unlike earlier puzzles of this type, the unwoven letters are provided but not placed.

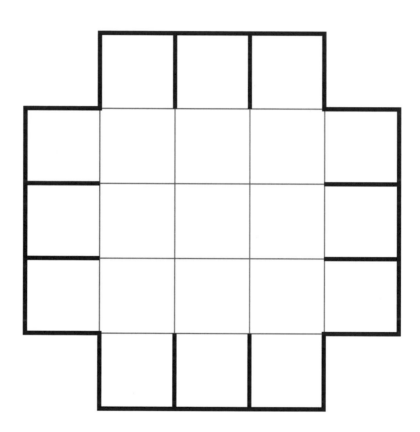

ACDDEFHRSTTW

Post-event

Task

Untethered

Work period

Sleepy

Value

Black Holes 6

Divide the grid into chunks along the guides provided so that each chunk contains one black hole, and so the digits in the chunk sum to the number in the black hole.

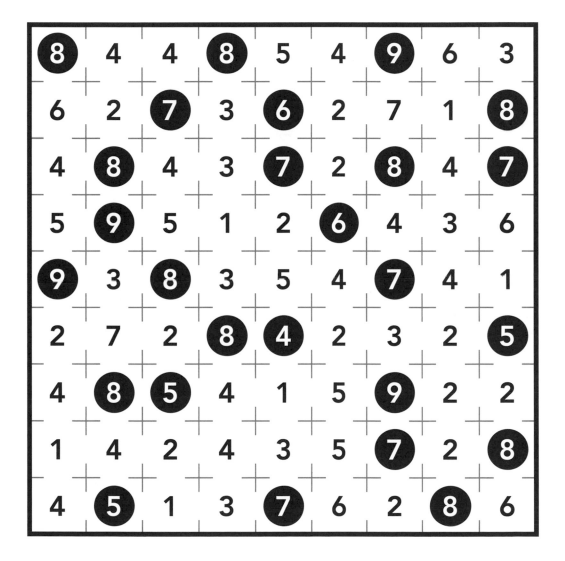

Numcross 10

Use the provided clues to fill the grid with numbers. No entry may start with a 0.

A	B	C		D	E		F	G
H				I			J	
		K	L		M	N		
	O			P		Q		
R				S	T			
U			V				W	X
		Y					Z	
	AA			BB	CC	DD		
EE			FF		GG			
HH			II	JJ		KK	LL	MM
NN			OO			PP		

Across

A. H across – 1

D. A down × 3

F. D across – 5

II. One-half of Y across

I. W across × 2

J. NN across + 1

K. Sum of the digits in S across

M. F down – 4000

O. BB across + 6000

Q. A perfect cube

R. LL down × 2

S. A palindrome

U. W across × 3

V. FF down × 3

W. T down – 1

Y. V across + W down

Z. T down + GG across

AA. X down + 1

BB. S across × 3

EE. AA down + 1000

GG. A perfect square

HH. Another perfect square

II. Y down – Y across

KK. NN across × OO across

NN. J across – 1

OO. NN across + 10

PP. JJ down × 9

Down

A. NN across × 2

B. L down + 3

C. O across + Y across

D. OO across × 3

E. Two-sevenths of M across

F. EE across + T down

G. N down – 1

L. W across × 5

N. R down × 2

O. L down × NN across

(Continued)

P. Contains one of each even digit

R. Another perfect cube

T. Another perfect square

V. Another perfect square

W. Z across × 2

X. Digits that sum to J across

Y. LL down × MM down

AA. Digits that sum to W across

CC. T down × 3

DD. EE down × 8

EE. Digits that sum to NN across

FF. F across × 2

JJ. MM down in reverse

LL. V down – 5

MM. One-third of X down

Slither Fence 4

Draw a fence connecting the left and right sides of the grid along the grid lines, with no breaks, loops, or forks in the fence line. Every square with a number must be surrounded by that many fence pieces.

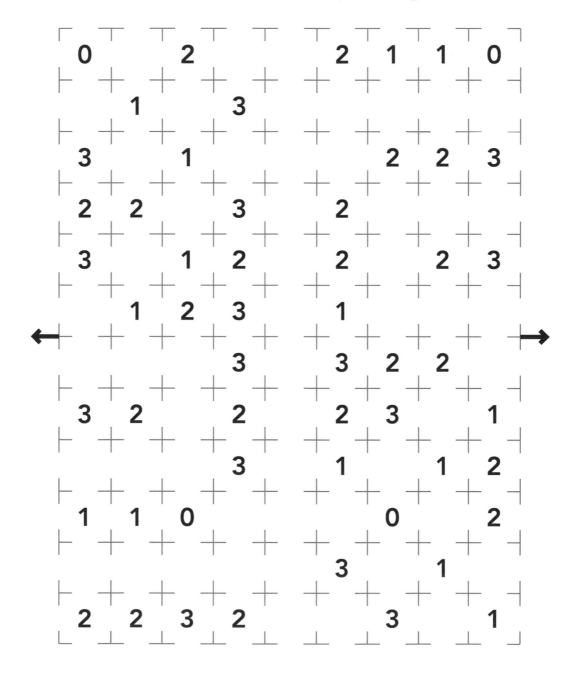

Penny Candy 5

Penny candy has gone up in price a fair bit. Use the total prices of the sets of four candies to figure out how much each piece of candy costs.

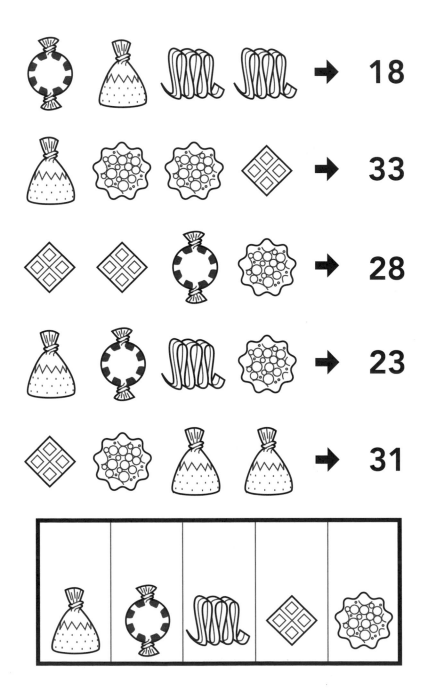

Rearrangement 9 & 10

Rearrange the letters in PREPPING SHOES to spell an occasion where someone would be doing a lot of walking around a mall.

Rearrange the letters in ARCTIC MUCK 'ERE to spell a set of wheels that specializes in something cold.

Word Funnel 8

Fill each section of the funnel with a six-letter word made up of the six letters above it. Clues have been provided in no particular order.

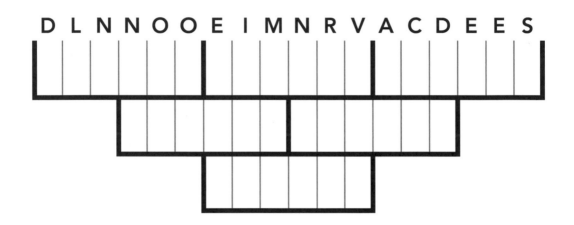

D L N N O O E I M N R V A C D E E S

Place to watch a movie

Stopped

Unwanted rodents

Seller or provider of services

Biggest city in England

Like some Scandinavians

Maze 4

Make your way from the top of the maze to the bottom.
(Or vice versa.)

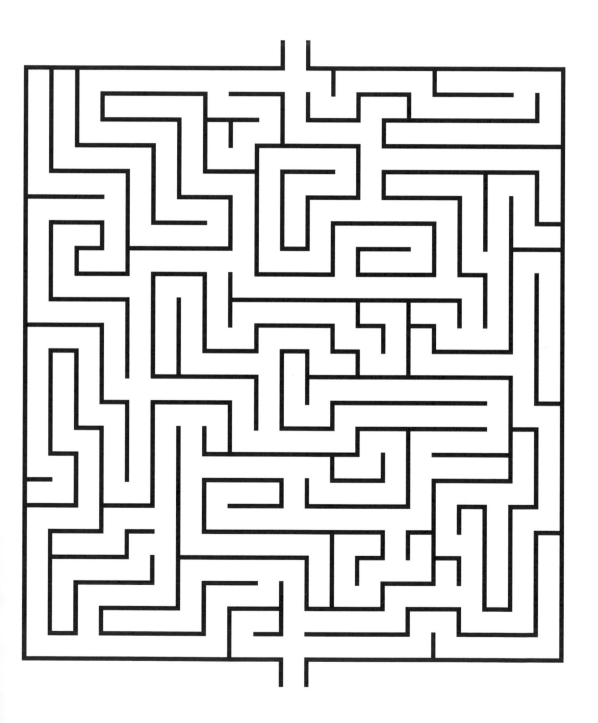

Woven Words 10

Use the clues to weave six words together in the grid below; three going across and three going down. Unlike earlier puzzles of this type, the unwoven letters are provided but not placed.

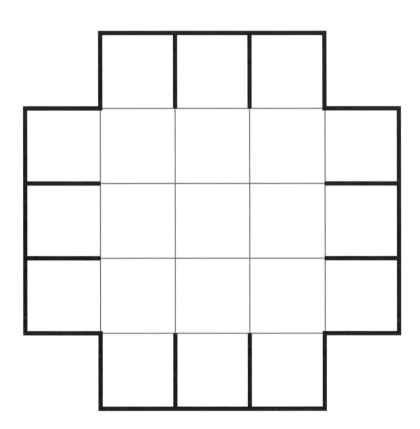

ABCCEEGKSSTV

Same

Simple

Mr. Gable or Mr. Kent

Complain

Passes over

Stop at

Cube Logic 10

Which of the four foldable patterns can be folded to make the block displayed?

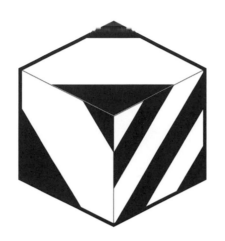

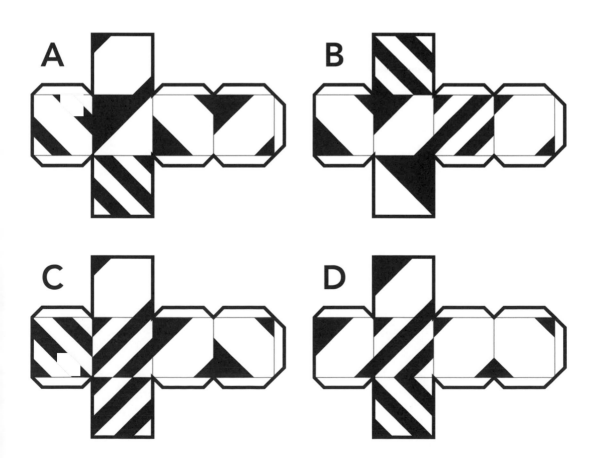

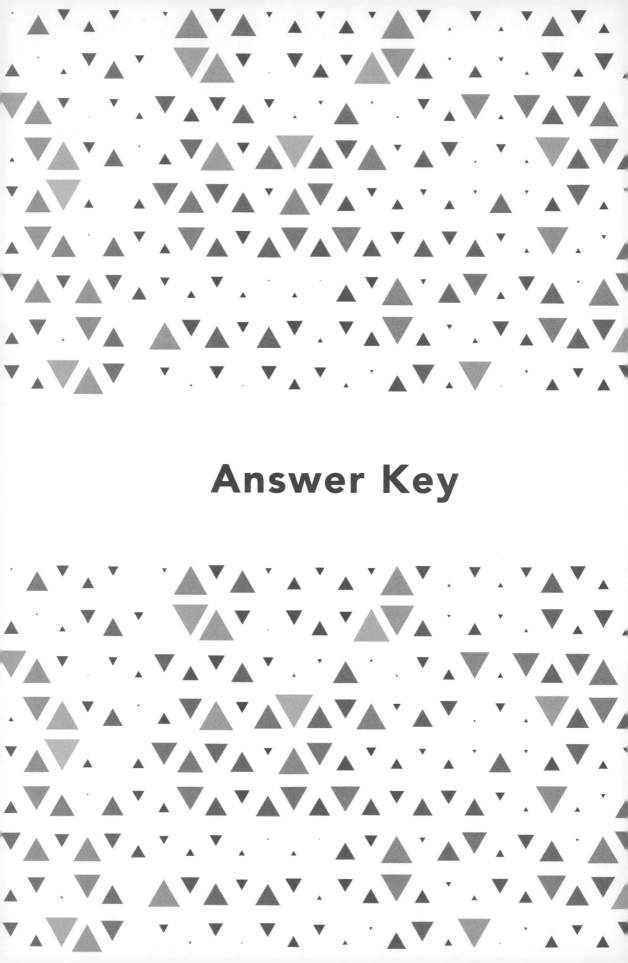

Answer Key

BLACK HOLES

Black Holes 1

```
5 9 2 7 2 4 5 9 2
7 4 3 4 8 2 2 3 2
2 3 4 2 2 9 5 1 7
5 4 1 5 4 4 2 3 5
2 1 4 1 3 3 5 1 5
6 1 2 6 2 9 3 7 1
8 8 3 7 5 4 3 2 4
3 5 6 4 5 3 5 8 2
2 4 2 3 8 2 7 6 1
```

Black Holes 2

```
7 8 4 7 3 6 4 2 2
1 4 5 3 7 5 2 3 1
5 1 5 9 4 5 9 5 4
3 4 8 1 8 1 3 2 7
2 6 3 3 9 2 1 5 1
7 2 2 4 9 3 4 1 2
2 5 7 1 2 6 7 8 1
8 1 1 6 7 4 5 5 2
6 3 7 2 2 7 3 6 8
```

Black Holes 3

```
4 2 7 5 7 2 5 9 2
7 5 2 8 2 8 2 2 3
3 2 8 3 6 4 3 6 10
1 7 6 5 4 2 9 8 5
3 5 3 7 9 8 3 3 2
2 1 4 5 5 2 9 6 2
8 1 5 9 7 3 4 2 4
6 7 2 4 8 9 5 1 4
1 3 8 4 1 7 2 3 7
```

Black Holes 4

```
5 4 8 2 4 1 2 8 5
7 2 5 2 1 7 6 3 8
2 10 2 5 6 2 5 2 4
8 5 7 8 3 6 3 4 7
9 1 6 3 3 9 7 3 1
5 7 2 6 3 5 1 8 4
4 3 5 7 1 4 4 2 5
2 5 2 10 3 1 9 3 9
9 7 8 2 6 4 4 9 6
```

Black Holes 5

```
7 1 6 7 1 3 2 5 9
6 4 9 5 5 8 1 8 3
1 3 3 1 6 4 1 9 6
6 5 7 4 1 5 6 3 8
2 6 4 8 5 1 3 8 2
4 5 8 5 6 7 2 5 6
5 3 2 3 9 1 8 2 7
2 6 1 4 3 8 4 4 3
4 2 4 7 3 1 3 6 3
```

Black Holes 6

```
8 4 4 8 5 4 9 6 3
6 2 7 3 6 2 7 1 8
4 8 4 3 7 2 8 4 7
5 9 5 1 2 6 4 3 6
9 3 8 3 5 4 7 4 1
2 7 2 8 4 2 3 2 5
4 8 5 4 1 5 9 2 2
1 4 2 4 3 5 7 2 8
4 5 1 3 7 6 2 8 6
```

CHESS SUM SUDOKU

Chess Sum Sudoku 1

Chess Sum Sudoku 2

Chess Sum Sudoku 3

Chess Sum Sudoku 4

Chess Sum Sudoku 5

CUBE LOGIC

1. A and F
2. A and C
3. B and D
4. A
5. D

6. C
7. A
8. D
9. B
10. C

FINDER'S FEE

$7891

A. u**SE VEN**tilators

B. w**EIGHT**lifting

C. macaro**NI NE**arly

D. b**ONE**

MAZES

Maze 1

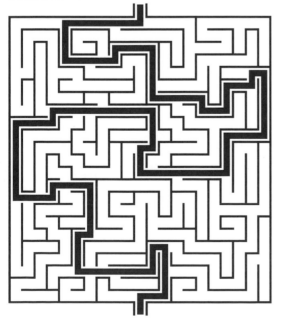

Maze 2

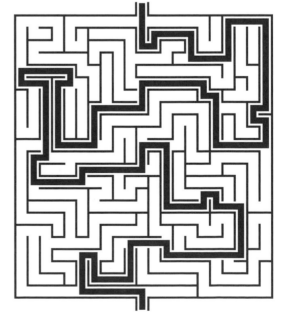

Maze 3

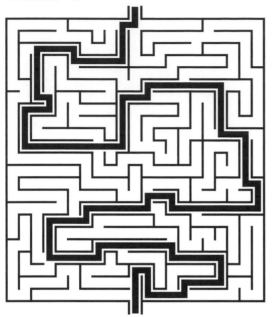

Maze 4

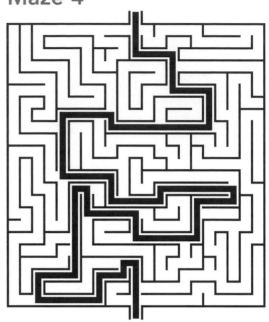

NO UNCERTAIN TERMS

NO Uncertain Terms 1
MIN**NO**W

CA**NO**E

E**NO**UGH

RE**NO**

NOTICE

NO Uncertain Terms 3
PI**NO**CCHIO

NOTARY

YOKO O**NO**

K**NO**WLEDGE

RE**NO**VATE

NO Uncertain Terms 2
NOVICE

PI**NO**T **NO**IR

S**NO**WMAN

K**NO**T

HO**NO**R

NO Uncertain Terms 4
VOLCA**NO**

LI**NO**LEUM

NORTHWEST

NORWAY

S**NO**B

NUMCROSS

Numcross 1

1	1	2	5	■	4	5
6	9	5	0	■	2	0
2	7	■	8	8	4	0
■	■	7	9	1	■	■
2	3	4	1	■	7	2
4	7	■	1	9	1	7
3	7	■	1	9	9	8

Numcross 2

3	8	9	■	■	6	3
1	6	1	6	■	1	2
■	■	2	4	8	6	0
■	2	7	■	6	1	■
7	4	5	8	0	■	■
7	5	■	1	2	4	3
8	4	■	■	4	2	6

Numcross 3

3	2	2	3	■	8	6
1	1	2	8	■	9	0
1	1	■	7	7	7	5
■	2	2	7	■	■	■
1	4	7	7	■	1	8
2	5	■	8	6	7	9
1	4	■	3	4	5	6

Numcross 4

5	6	■	■	1	6	9
4	4	1	■	1	4	4
■	■	3	2	■	2	4
■	2	0	6	4	8	■
1	5	■	4	9	■	■
9	8	3	■	6	1	1
5	1	1	■	■	3	6

Numcross 5

5	1	3	■	3	1	5
1	0	1	■	1	0	2
■	■	6	4	■	2	9
■	2	2	5	2	5	■
4	1	■	6	9	■	■
5	0	2	■	2	5	2
1	0	5	■	9	0	1

Numcross 6

1	7	1	■	3	4	1
1	7	9	■	1	0	6
■	■	8	1	■	5	0
■	2	8	6	4	0	■
1	0	■	2	7	■	■
4	3	2	■	7	4	5
6	8	2	■	4	0	4

Numcross 7

1	2	■	1	2	5	■	■	1	7
2	0	■	4	5	1	■	■	1	1
4	1	2	5	■	4	1	4	5	■
3	4	3	■	2	4	2	■	■	■
■	■	1	5	0	■	1	6	2	■
1	8	■	9	6	9	■	4	1	■
5	1	2	■	8	6	1	■	■	■
■	■	6	5	4	■	8	9	1	■
1	3	0	1	■	1	7	1	5	■
4	7	■	7	5	0	■	1	3	■
3	5	■	1	1	9	■	1	6	■

Numcross 8

9	6	3	■	1	7	■	3	1	■
1	4	4	■	8	2	■	1	0	■
■	■	7	2	■	9	9	9	3	■
■	1	9	5	1	■	9	3	■	■
6	0	■	■	7	2	0	■	■	■
2	7	■	3	3	3	■	8	1	■
■	■	3	6	9	■	■	2	6	■
■	1	2	■	5	4	5	4	■	■
8	4	1	5	■	9	3	■	■	■
7	5	■	6	9	■	4	3	4	■
9	8	■	1	5	■	7	0	4	■

Numcross 9

7	4	■	1	7	1	■	5	1	■
4	7	■	1	5	0	■	1	1	■
1	1	1	1	■	1	2	7	9	■
6	3	8	■	3	0	0	■	■	■
■	■	1	2	1	■	1	2	5	■
7	2	■	7	9	2	■	2	5	■
3	0	3	■	7	1	1	■	■	■
■	■	3	1	5	■	6	1	1	■
1	8	0	9	■	1	8	8	3	■
1	5	■	6	6	0	■	6	1	■
5	7	■	6	7	1	■	1	0	■

Numcross 10

2	7	9	■	6	6	■	6	1	■
2	8	0	■	3	0	■	1	2	■
■	■	1	7	■	2	1	0	7	■
■	8	4	5	4	■	2	7	■	■
6	2	■	■	8	1	8	■	■	■
4	5	■	3	6	6	■	1	5	■
■	■	5	6	0	■	■	9	7	■
■	5	8	■	2	4	5	4	■	■
6	0	9	1	■	8	1	■	■	■
4	9	■	2	9	■	2	3	1	■
1	1	■	2	1	■	8	1	9	■

PENNY CANDY

Penny Candy 1

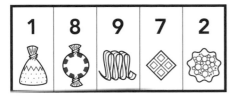

Penny Candy 2

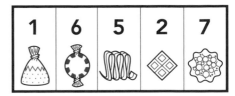

Penny Candy 3

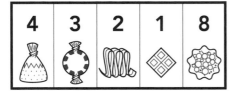

Penny Candy 4

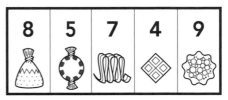

Penny Candy 5

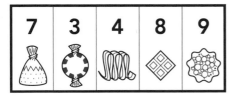

REARRANGEMENT

1. Old-School Diner
2. A Fishing Trip
3. Footlong Sub
4. Holiday Party
5. Prank Phone Call
6. Garden Shears
7. Logging Road
8. Grocery Bag
9. Shopping Spree
10. Ice Cream Truck

ROWS GARDEN

Rows Garden 1

```
      V I D
Y O G I N E V E R
T R U E A N I S E
G L O B E I R I S
S E V E N A Y E S
E R A S E T R O T
T I N T N E E D S
      I L L
```

Rows Garden 2

```
      S I D
T A I L A N V I L
E D N A B E I N G
S U R F F L O O D
H E D G E I D L E
S T O R E G L A D
A P R I L F R E D
      P R E
```

Rows Garden 3

```
      C H A
B O S S R I V E R
N O T E I N E R T
M I N C E S T A R
B L E N D D R A T
R I D E F E V E R
B E G A N S O R T
      R E W
```

Rows Garden 4

```
      L O W
A N G L E F O L D
T E L L C R A N E
T R E E V E N O M
S T A R A I S L E
C R E E D L O R E
S M A L L R I C H
      A C E
```

Rows Garden 5

```
      C A R
A I R E D T A L K
P E R U N I X O N
S E P T E M B E R
C I T Y G R A T E
B A L S A E V I L
R E L I C K I N G
      T E L
```

SLITHER FENCE

Slither Fence 1

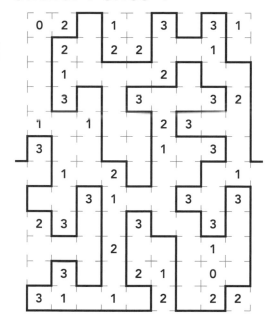

Slither Fence 2

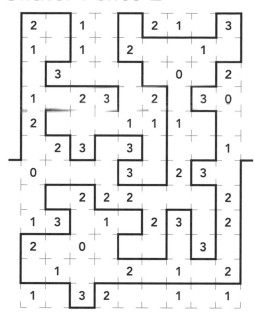

Slither Fence 3

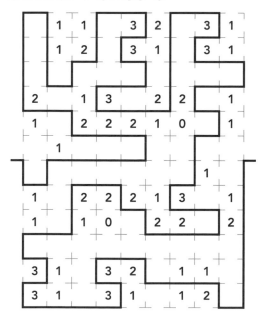

Slither Fence 4

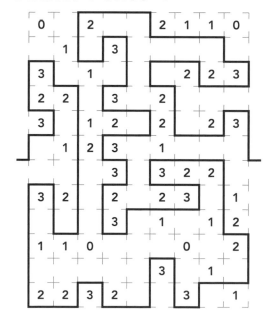

SUDOKU TV

Sudoku TV 1

```
H Y D A P S
S A P H D Y
D S H P Y A
A P Y S H D
P D A Y S H
Y H S D A P
```

Sudoku TV 2

```
T L A K M O C
O C M T K L A
L K O A C T M
M A T L O C K
C T K M L A O
A M C O T K L
K O L C A M T
```

Sudoku TV 3

```
N G R A T D E
T E N D G R A
A T G E R N D
D R A G N E T
E N D T A G R
G A E R D T N
R D T N E A G
```

Sudoku TV 4

```
N K Y I C A E D V
A V E N D Y K I C
D I C K E V N Y A
C Y A D K E I V N
K D I V A N C E Y
V E N Y I C D A K
I A V C N D Y K E
E C K A Y I V N D
Y N D E V K A C I
```

Sudoku TV 5

```
D A H B C R Y N U
C U N Y A H R B D
B R Y U N D A H C
H B A D Y N C U R
U N D C R A H Y B
R Y C H B U N D A
A D R N U Y B C H
Y C U A H B D R N
N H B R D C U A Y
```

THROWING SHADE

Throwing Shade 1

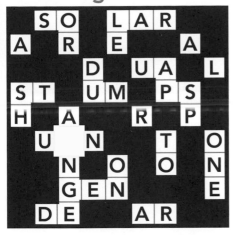

Throwing Shade 2

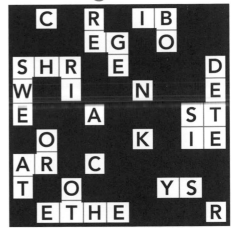

Throwing Shade 3

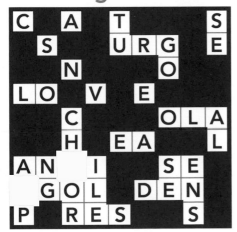

Throwing Shade 4

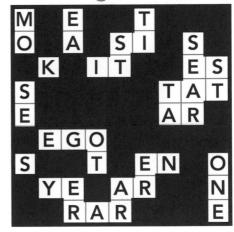

Throwing Shade 5

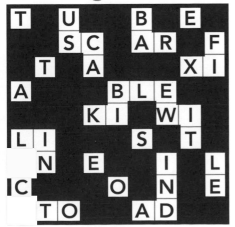

TRANSIT MAP

Transit Map 1

Southbound

:00	Camera
:06	Clam
:10	Sides
:15	Organ
:20	Sleep
:25	

Northbound

:25	Peel
:29	Snag
:33	Rose
:37	Dismal
:43	Care
:47	Mac
:50	

Transit Map 2

Southbound

:00	Sew
:03	Older
:08	Obey
:12	Ed
:14	Erode
:19	Remotes
:26	On
:28	

Northbound

:28	Nose
:32	Tome
:36	Redo
:40	Red Eye
:46	Bored
:51	Lowes
:56	

Transit Map 3

Southbound

:00	Deli
:04	Ample
:09	Hell
:13	Ebb
:16	Urge
:20	Roger
:25	If
:27	

Northbound

:27	Fire
:31	Gore
:35	Grub
:39	Belle
:44	Help
:48	Mailed
:54	

Transit Map 4

Southbound

:00	Native
:06	Looms
:11	Sample
:17	Hoot
:21	Embark
:27	

Northbound

:27	Krab
:31	Me Too
:36	Help
:40	Mass
:44	Moo
:47	Levi
:51	Tan
:54	

Transit Map 5

Southbound

:00	Donut
:05	Utter
:10	Cessna
:16	Vote
:20	Kite
:24	Yam
:27	

Northbound

:27	Ma
:29	Yeti
:33	Keto
:37	Vans
:41	Secret
:47	Tutu
:51	Nod
:54	

Transit Map 6

Southbound

:00	Spine
:05	Lump
:09	Amigo
:14	Yore
:18	Hate
:22	Brood
:27	

Northbound

:27	Door
:31	Beta
:35	Hero
:39	Yogi
:43	Map
:46	Mule
:50	Nips
:54	

Transit Map 7

Southbound

:00
    Wart
:04
    Spin
:08
    Tacos
:13
    Impact
:19
    Celeste
:26

Northbound

:26
    ETs
:29
    Elect
:34
    Cap
:37
    Miso
:41
    Catnip
:47
    Straw
:52

Transit Map 8

Southbound

:00
    Motel
:05
    Fire
:09
    Sonnet
:15
    Foil
:19
    Aces
:23
    Rap
:26

Northbound

:26
    Parse
:31
    Cali
:35
    Often
:40
    Nose
:44
    Rifle
:49
    Tom
:52

WORD FUNNEL

Word Funnel 1

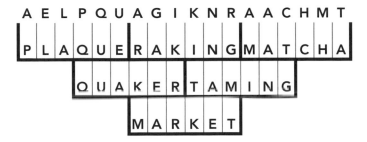

Word Funnel 2

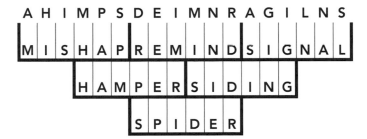

Word Funnel 3

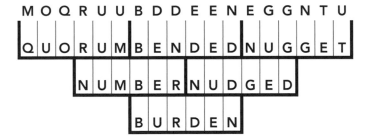

Word Funnel 4

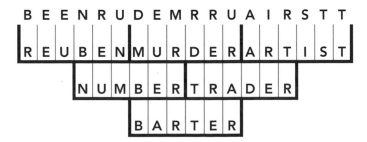

Word Funnel 5

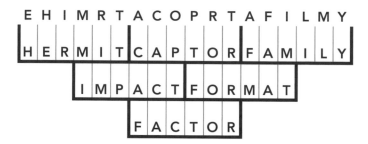

```
E H I M R T A C O P R T A F I L M Y
H E R M I T C A P T O R F A M I L Y
    I M P A C T F O R M A T
        F A C T O R
```

Word Funnel 6

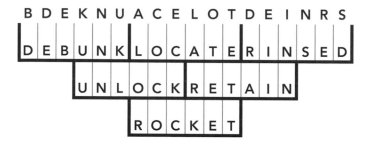

```
B D E K N U A C E L O T D E I N R S
D E B U N K L O C A T E R I N S E D
    U N L O C K R E T A I N
        R O C K E T
```

Word Funnel 7

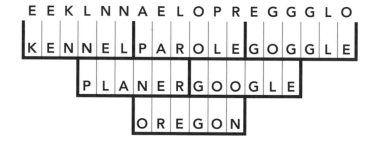

```
E E K L N N A E L O P R E G G G L O
K E N N E L P A R O L E G O G G L E
    P L A N E R G O O G L E
        O R E G O N
```

Word Funnel 8

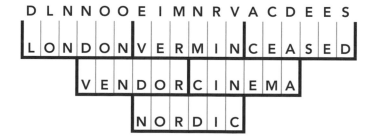

```
D L N N O O E I M N R V A C D E E S
L O N D O N V E R M I N C E A S E D
    V E N D O R C I N E M A
        N O R D I C
```

WOVEN WORDS

Woven Words 1

```
    W B S
  S E A T S
  B A S E S
  A V I A N
    E L L
```

Woven Words 2

```
    E S T
  E X T R A
  W I R E S
  A S I A N
    T P D
```

Woven Words 3

```
    S C N
  O T H E R
  B R O W N
  H A R E S
    W E R
```

Woven Words 4

```
    S C C
  S T O R M
  F E R A L
  B R A V O
    N L E
```

Woven Words 5

```
    S S F
  T U L I P
  A G I L E
  S A M M Y
    R E S
```

Woven Words 6

```
    R A S
  M O L A R
  A B O U T
  P I N T O
    N E E
```

Woven Words 7

```
    S G C
B E R R Y
S P O U T
D I V E R
  A E L
```

Woven Words 8

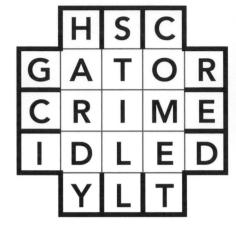

```
    H S C
G A T O R
C R I M E
I D L E D
  Y L T
```

Woven Words 9

```
  S W F
C H O R E
T I R E D
A F T E R
  T H D
```

Woven Words 10

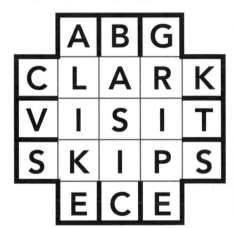

```
  A B G
C L A R K
V I S I T
S K I P S
  E C E
```

Exercise Your Mind at American Mensa®

At American Mensa, we love puzzles. In fact, we have events—large and small—centered around games and puzzles.

Of course, with tens of thousands of members from ages 2 to 102, we are much more than that. Our one shared trait might be one you share, too: high intelligence, measured in the top 2 percent of the general public in a standardized test.

Get-togethers with other Mensans—from small pizza nights up to larger events like our annual Mind Games®—are always stimulating and fun. Roughly 130 Special Interest Groups (we call them SIGs) offer the best of the real and virtual worlds. Highlighting the Mensa newsstand is our award-winning magazine, *Mensa Bulletin*, which stimulates the curious mind with unique features that add perspective to our fast-paced world.

Then there are the practical benefits of membership, such as exclusive offers through our partners and member discounts on magazine subscriptions, online shopping, and financial services.

Find out how to qualify or take our practice test at americanmensa.org/join.

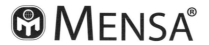